Recipes for the
Specific Carbohydrate Diet™

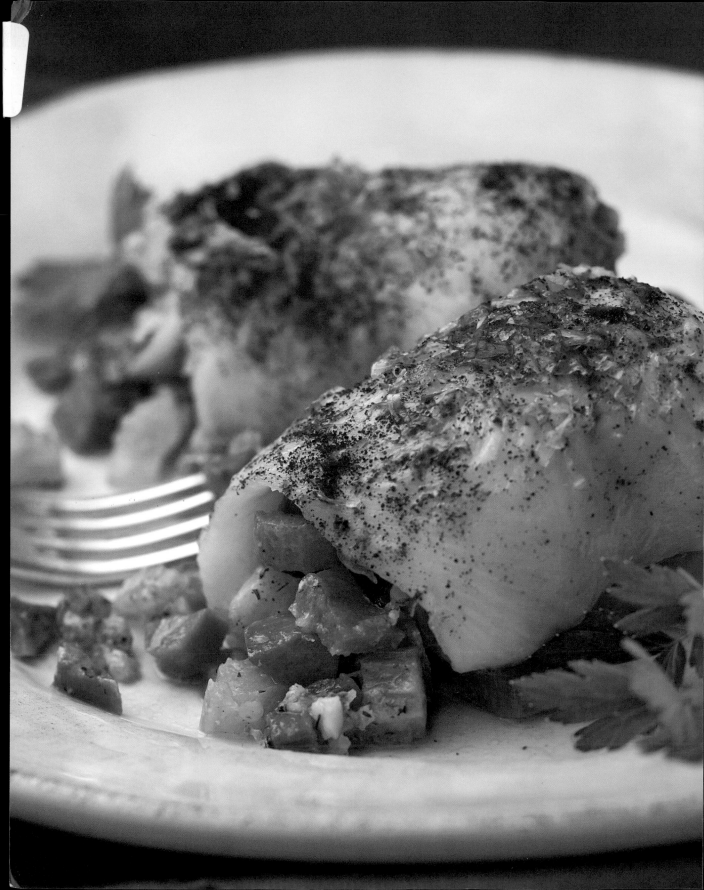

Recipes for the
Specific Carbohydrate Diet™

The Grain-Free, Lactose-Free, Sugar-Free Solution to IBD,
Celiac Disease, Autism, Cystic Fibrosis,
and Other Health Conditions

Raman Prasad

with Niloufer Moochhala

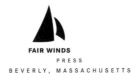

FAIR WINDS
PRESS
BEVERLY, MASSACHUSETTS

DEDICATION

*To our families, for the good meals and memories
that we have captured in this book.*

Text ©2008 Raman Prasad
Photography ©2008 Rockport Publishers

First published in the USA in 2008 by
Fair Winds Press, a member of
Quayside Publishing Group
100 Cummings Center
Suite 406-L
Beverly, MA 01915-6101
www.fairwindspress.com

17 16 15 14 13   11 12 13 14

ISBN-13: 978-1-59233-282-3
ISBN-10: 1-59233-282-X

Library of Congress Cataloging-in-Publication Data

Prasad, Raman.
  Recipes for the specific carbohydrate diet / by Raman Prasad; with Niloufer Moochhala.
     p. cm.
  Includes index.
  ISBN-13: 978-1-59233-282-3
  ISBN-10: 1-59233-282-X
 1. Inflammatory bowel diseases--Diet therapy--Recipes. 2. Carbohydrate intolerance--Diet
therapy--Recipes. I. Moochhala, Niloufer. II. Title.
  RC862.I53P73 2007
  641.5'6383--dc22
                                    2007032781

Cover design: Howard Grossman
Book layout: Leslie Haimes
Photography: Glenn Scott

Printed and bound in China

The information in this book is for educational purposes only. It is not intended to replace
the advice of a physician or medical practitioner. Please see your health care provider before
beginning any new health program.

Specific Carbohydrate Diet and SCD are trademarks of Kirkton Press Limited.

Contents

Foreword

My name is Raquel Nieves, I am a pediatrician, and I have Crohn's disease.

My symptoms began in high school and progressed for years until I dropped down to 82 pounds, suffering from daily fevers, severe abdominal pain, fatigue, and anemia. Subsequent standard medications provided little relief and caused many side effects.

I came across Elaine Gottschall's book, *Breaking the Vicious Cycle*, which detailed the Specific Carbohydrate Diet (SCD)™, while in medical school in 2001.

The diet completely gave me my life back. It worked beyond my imagination and within a month, I significantly improved. Within a few months, I was completely off of all medications.

Meanwhile, excited and completely surprised over how well the SCD worked, I told my doctor about it. Unfortunately, the idea of a diet was met with a lot of resistance. He told me that I was making a mistake, and that it wasn't the diet that had helped me improve, but that it was just spontaneous remission. Knowing that Crohn's is a relapsing and remitting disease, he said my symptoms would return if I did not take the medications they were recommending. Because I was in the medical field, I was devastated that my colleagues did not believe or even want to consider dietary therapy.

This skepticism is what led me, along with Roger Jackson, M.D., to publish a medical paper entitled *Specific Carbohydrate Diet in the Treatment of Inflammatory Bowel Disease* in 2004. The paper discussed our Internet survey of 51 people who suffered from either Crohn's disease or ulcerative colitis—84 percent of whom were in remission since beginning the SCD. Of these, 61 percent were off all of their medications.

Being a doctor, I still do not understand why an alternative therapy such as a healthy diet is so threatening. Despite this trend, some doctors *have* begun to understand the relevance of the SCD and are investigating it, although funding has been difficult. Because this diet has helped me so immensely—and I know that I would not be a doctor today if I didn't adhere to it—I feel it is my duty to continue to advocate and press the medical community to at least investigate it further. My hope for this diet in the future is that it becomes one of the first-line treatments for inflammatory bowel disease (IBD). If research proves it to be effective, it should be offered as a treatment option, either alone or in conjunction with medications.

The best model I can compare this to would be in the case with diabetes. Research has shown how effective diet can be in managing diabetes. Doctors recommend and teach dietary modification to all of their diabetic patients. In addition, diet is used in conjunction with other standard medications unless diet alone controls the disorder. My hope is that one day the SCD will play this type of role in the treatment of IBD. The challenge to this diet, however, is that it requires strict adherence to be effective. Thankfully, Raman Prasad's creative recipes provide tasty meals that make the diet much easier to follow. They are culturally diverse, easy to make, and delicious.

Those of us on the SCD appreciate Raman Prasad and all of his efforts to restore health, well-being, and hope to all those suffering from IBD and similar diseases.

— Raquel Nieves, M.D.

Introduction

This book came into being due to a toothbrush I innocently swished in the Rio Grande River during a high school canoe trip and a resulting case of Montezuma's revenge. The incident led to months of antibiotics and antiparasitic medication, painful medical complications, and a diagnosis of ulcerative colitis at age seventeen.

During a five-minute, post-sigmoidoscopy meeting on the day I was diagnosed, a gastroenterologist quickly told me, "Do not eat raw vegetables, fruit, popcorn, or nuts ever again." I was given a prescription for prednisone, and life veered off for a while. Years eighteen through twenty-three passed by in a surreal blur. I could never count on feeling well the next day.

At age twenty-four, after a hospital stay and with drugs having little effect on the disease, the doctor described my intestines as resembling "bloody hamburger." Surgery was the next option, and hope waned.

Another Chance

However, that same year, I was lucky enough to find Elaine Gottschall's book *Breaking the Vicious Cycle* through the soon-to-be-popular Internet (it was 1996). The book proposed treating inflammatory bowel disease (IBD), diverticulitis, celiac disease, cystic fibrosis, and chronic diarrhea through a "Specific Carbohydrate Diet (SCD)™." After reading it twice, the premise behind the diet made sense.

The author described a "vicious cycle" in which injury to the surface of the small intestine leads to the inability to properly digest the carbohydrates in many foods, including bread, pasta, rice, and milk. When the body cannot digest these foods, the undigested carbohydrates become energy that fuels bacterial overgrowth in the intestinal tract. The small intestine becomes injured further and responds to the increase of bacterial by-products by creating more mucus. In turn, the mucus leads to impaired digestion and the cycle escalates, resulting in symptoms such as diarrhea and eventually IBD.

The diet attempts to break this cycle by avoiding carbohydrates that cannot be properly digested, thereby depriving harmful bacteria of energy. In addition, the diet includes acidophilus, obtained through homemade yogurt, which restores the intestine's bacterial balance.

The premise was clear, but the diet certainly seemed tough: no rice, no bread, no potatoes, no *too many things*. However, once IBD symptoms (diarrhea, blood, and cramping) subside,* fruits and vegetables—foods I rarely ate with ulcerative colitis—can gradually be re-introduced to the diet. Many years had passed since I had dared to eat a salad.

So I decided to give the diet a try. I emptied out my apartment of "illegal" foods and stocked up on SCD "legal" ones at the grocery store. (See the chart on page 17 for examples of "legal" and "illegal" foods.)

At first it was difficult to tell whether the diet was working. I was on the steroid prednisone, which hid any pain and stopped diarrhea, but also left me feeling numb and confused. After six weeks, however, a notable change came in the form of a blood test for the liver: instead of my typical "abnormally high" result, the test came back normal—and a liver biopsy was cancelled. Shortly after, I began weaning myself off the steroids, which took nearly six months, but my bowel movements had become normal, and the pain in my abdomen was gone. As the months passed and my energy returned, I felt strong again, and best of all, I dared to look ahead and make future plans—plans that included going back to school for graduate studies and then finding a job in New York City. During this time I continued to read postings on an online SCD mailing list and, in 1999, I was able to use a lull at work to organize recipes from the SCD mailings and post them at www.scdrecipe.com.

Meeting Elaine Gottschall

In the fall of 2001, Elaine Gottschall visited the New York metro area to make presentations in Brooklyn and Long Island. Eager to meet the woman responsible for giving me my life back, I took the Long Island Railroad out to a restaurant in Port Jefferson, New York, to attend a twenty-person brunch in Elaine's honor.

*NOTE: The diet appears to work for more than 80 percent of people who follow it strictly.[1] A rule of thumb is to try it for one month; some improvement usually appears after the third week. However, the variation in cases is fairly wide, depending on how ill the person is.

From her picture in *Breaking the Vicious Cycle*, I imagined Elaine, then eighty years old, as warm and soft-spoken. At 5-foot 8-inches, she was warm and kind, but she exuded the energy of someone half her age. (For the record, she wasn't soft-spoken, but had a strong, clear voice.) Her knowledge, as well as her humor, impressed us all that afternoon.

Over the years, I saw Elaine a number of times, helping at her SCD table during several conferences. The last time I saw Elaine was a few weeks before she passed away from cancer in September 2005, when I visited her near her home in Canada, a short trip outside of Toronto. (Mere months earlier, at age eighty-four, she had accompanied her young granddaughter on a transatlantic flight to Paris.)

Elaine had helped so many people with the SCD along the way, that now, in her time of need, there was an infinite number of people looking out for her. During my visit, people I had never met, but whose lives had been changed by the diet, warmly took me into their homes and fed me SCD meals. One woman prepared a vegetable-laden chicken soup to nourish Elaine in the small, comfortable Canadian hospital where she was staying.

Walking toward her hospital room, we were all filled with great sadness. But even in her pain, she was in good humor; on the subject of the diet, however, she became grave and concerned. She did not want her work to fall into disuse—she knew that for each person she had helped, there were hundreds more suffering. She simply asked us to keep the SCD alive.

All of us who have been helped by her work and who met her in person have done what we can—from opening clinics and consulting on the diet to simply passing along the name of her book. For me, what stands out the most is her selflessness, commitment, and perseverance. Even while she was in the hospital, I remember her taking a phone call so that she could help someone else who was ill.

This book is a small contribution to keep her work going. Realizing all that has been cooked for me over the past years, I feel increasingly appreciative of all the people around me—family, friends, and other fellow SCDers. I hope that in sharing these recipes, these feelings and good health are passed on to others.

In this book, we'll be traveling to many places. In the kitchen, we'll be cutting, mixing, baking, whirring, stirring, and tasting. Pushing our carts through the supermarket, we'll read labels and find SCD-safe foods. As we explore the book's varied recipes, we'll travel to different continents and see what they have to offer for the SCD diet. We'll also explore food for the holidays (there's no need to feel left out at these meals!). But before moving forward, let's first step back.

A Short History of the SCD

The SCD did not start recently. It wasn't developed with the motivation of making money, nor is it based on wishful thinking.

The diet's origins go back at least 120 years to the observations of Dr. Samuel Gee, who, in 1888, published a report titled *On the Celiac Affection*, in which he described patients with an intolerance to starchy foods, including rice and corn flour.[2] Elaine Gottschall was fond of quoting one of his lines: "We must never forget that what the patient takes beyond his power of digestion does harm."

Let's pick up the story in the 1920s. At the time, Dr. Sidney Valentine Haas, a Columbia University–educated physician, was working as a pediatrician in New York City. During his first decades of work, he saw many cases of celiac disease, many of which resulted in death (in the early 1900s, 25 percent of celiac patients died of the disease;[3] they simply could not digest many foods).

Through the course of his practice, Dr. Haas found that children with celiac disease could tolerate fruits, certain vegetables, and milk protein.[4] At the beginning of treatment, he started with bananas—ripe bananas with black spots on the skin. In 1924, Dr. Haas publicized his findings, and his dietary protocol soon became a standard for celiac disease.

An example of the prevalence of Dr. Haas' celiac diet may be found in the newspaper archives of *The New York Times*. During 1942, in the midst of World War II, the military requisitioned many merchant ships to transport supplies. This included ships normally used for transporting bananas into the United States and so resulted a banana shortage. To help reassure families with celiac patients who depended upon these bananas, *The New York Times* printed a letter by Dr. Haas, an excerpt of which appears below:

> "Among families having cases of celiac disease, there is considerable anxiety over the possibility of being unable to procure bananas for such cases.
>
> "As the originator of the modern banana treatment of this disease, I am being daily approached in regard to the problem … The United Fruit Company is doing all that is possible to meet the situation and any case of celiac disease can obtain bananas if available by addressing the United Fruit Company, Pier 3, North River.
>
> "Should a real banana famine occur, the government would doubtless cooperate with the banana companies to transport by air."[5]

Sidney V. Haas, M.D.
New York, August 4, 1942

In 1951, after treating more than 603 children with celiac disease—370 cases of which were studied intensely—Dr. Haas cured more than 98 percent of them. He published his findings in the 1951 medical book The Management of Celiac Disease. In that book, Dr. Haas refers to his protocol as the "Specific Carbohydrate Diet."

Elaine Gottschall Meets Dr. Haas

In 1960, Judy Gottschall, age eight, suffered from severe ulcerative colitis. After three years of seemingly endless visits to the doctor, her health continued to deteriorate and ultimately led to the scheduling of surgery to remove part of her intestine.

Prior to the surgery, her mother, Elaine Gottschall, feeling heartbroken, began to cry. At this moment, one of the doctors reportedly asked her why she was crying and then said to her, "You're the one who did this to your daughter." (During that time period, one popular psychiatric theory held mothers responsible for causing ulcerative colitis.)

Tired, upset, and angry, Elaine instead took Judy and went back home. That night, one of Elaine's friends came to offer comfort. On her way to Elaine's home, the friend spoke to an acquaintance who knew someone with similar digestive problems—problems cured by a "Dr. Haas."

After hearing the news, Elaine tracked down Dr. Haas, who was, of course, Dr. Sidney Valentine Haas. As Elaine described it in a 2003 e-mail, posted on www.scdiet.org:

> *"We found him at the age of 90, his gray hair pinned back with a bobby pin, working away in his mahogany-paneled office on Park Avenue and 91st Street, New York City, after three years of fruitless searching for an answer for Judy, stricken with [ulcerative colitis] and horrendous night seizures resembling schizophrenic seizures.*
>
> *"He was the first of 15 doctors to ask me 'What is your child eating?'"*

Dr. Haas instructed Elaine and Judy on how to treat the ulcerative colitis using the Specific Carbohydrate Diet. Judy's symptoms of night terrors disappeared almost immediately. Digestive improvement came slowly but steadily. Eighteen months later, Judy was greatly improved and on her way to recovery.

In the years afterward, when Elaine Gottschall heard of other mothers with similarly ill children, she told them of Dr. Haas and the SCD.

In December 1964, four years after first treating Judy, Dr. Haas passed away. In his obituary, *The New York Times* described Dr. Haas' celiac treatment as having saved "uncounted lives." However, time and treatment had moved on. Preferring medication instead of diet, doctors no longer asked, "What is your child eating?"

Dr. Haas' son Merrill continued his father's practice, but as the years passed, Dr. Haas' knowledge faded from collective memory. It would have sat unused, buried in university libraries had Elaine not let it go. The more suffering she saw, the more it bothered her. Finally, her husband Herb, sharing her thoughts and always fully supportive, said she had to go out there and "find out what the blankety-blank was going on."

Taking it upon herself to help IBD sufferers, Elaine returned to school to learn why the diet worked. Not having taken a class since 1939, she returned to school at the age of forty-seven to brush up on high school math. After completing this step, Elaine realized that to continue undergraduate and graduate studies would take many years—but she would not falter from her goal.

In 1973, she earned her undergraduate degree in biology. She then focused her attention on the digestive tract, spending a year at Rutgers University Department of Graduate Studies in Nutrition. Following this, she went on to earn her Master's degree in biochemistry from the University of Western Ontario, where she conducted further investigation into the changes that occur in the bowel wall in inflammatory bowel disease.

All of this time, Elaine had a copy of Dr. Haas' 1951 book, *The Management of Celiac Disease*. In the last chapter of the book, Dr. Haas uses precise, Sherlock Holmesian–logic to suggest a cause of the disease. With more modern research tools and recent studies available, Elaine took this hypothesis and "reverse-engineered" the diet, coming to a better understanding of how and why the diet worked.

Writing Her Own Book

Elaine started personally assisting many people with the diet. Simultaneously, she set out to write what she had learned. In 1987, she completed work on a book titled *Food and the Gut Reaction*. In it she described the mechanisms that perpetuate IBD, celiac disease, diverticulitis, and cystic fibrosis, as well as how to use the SCD diet to heal the intestine and return the body to a healthy state. The first half of the book explained how to implement the diet and the science behind it, and the second half contained recipes.

In two years, it sold 200 copies. However, Elaine, by then a Canadian resident, continued to speak vigorously about the diet and was invited to appear on the *Dini Petty Show*, the Canadian version of *Oprah*. Elaine's segment ran for eight minutes on national TV. In the next ten days, 23,000 copies of the book were sold and word began to spread. In 1994, she republished the book under the name *Breaking the Vicious Cycle*. Since that time, the book has continued to be a best seller, has been translated into six languages, and has helped thousands of people.

The Rationale Behind the SCD

During IBD, the state of the intestine resembles the aftermath of a major hurricane. So many things are going wrong that it's difficult to know where to start. These include:

- **Injured Intestinal Lining.** The cells of the small intestine, where food molecules are further broken down by enzymes and then absorbed by the body, have been injured. This means that the enzymes at the ends of these cells are not available to break down particular types of complex carbohydrates, such as those in bread, rice, and soy.

- **Bacterial Overgrowth.** When carbohydrates are not broken down, they serve as an energy source for harmful bacteria. As these bacteria feed (ferment) on the undigested carbohydrates, they produce by-products of gas and acid, which further damage the intestinal lining. Also, as these bacteria feed, they multiply.

- **Mucus Secretion.** To protect itself against acids and other bacterial by-products, the intestinal lining produces mucus. However, in attempting to block harmful substances, the mucus also stops digestive enzymes from coming into contact with undigested carbohydrate molecules. Again, this leaves more undigested carbohydrates, leading to more bacterial overgrowth.

- **Malabsorption.** With the combination of intestinal injury and mucus secretion, the intestine cannot properly absorb food, further weakening the body.

- **Immune Response.** In an effort to stop the intestinal chaos, the intestinal cells start producing tumor necrosis factor, or TNF, which signals the body's inflammatory response. This is the "autoimmune" response in conditions such as Crohn's disease. (Recent investigations show that certain types of beneficial bacteria, or probiotics, trigger a change in the intestinal mucosa, and the mucosal cells reduce their TNF production.)[6]

- **Leaky Gut (Increased Intestinal Permeability).** The intestinal wall is made up of tightly bound cells that block damaging substances from passing into the body. However, in the midst of this chaos, openings start to develop between the cells, allowing potentially harmful substances to pass through. A 2005 study noted that increased intestinal permeability has a "primary role" in the development of ulcerative colitis and Crohn's disease.[7] The study also noted that intestinal permeability appears to precede the onset of IBD.

When food is eaten in this state, it feeds the storm. Specifically, undigested carbohydrates provide more bacterial fuel, strengthening all the negative events listed above.

The SCD attempts to heal the intestine through a two-pronged approach:

1. Removing foods that feed harmful bacteria and cannot be digested by the injured intestine. In particular, the injured intestine has trouble breaking down specific types of carbohydrates.

2. Restoring the balance of beneficial bacteria, by using probiotics, primarily in the form of homemade yogurt.

This approach slowly "starves out" the harmful bacteria, stopping mucus production, down-regulating inflammation, restoring the balance of beneficial intestinal flora, and giving the intestine a chance to heal.

When Elaine described this process in her 1986 publication *Food and the Gut Reaction*, gastroenterologists took little notice of the role of intestinal bacteria/flora and probiotics in inflammatory bowel disease. Even more recently, in 2000, the concisely written book *Understanding Crohn's Disease and Colitis*, which summarized IBD knowledge of that time, only mentioned probiotics in two sentences. These sentences appear in the last chapter, on the last page, right before a half-page description of using nicotine for IBD treatment.

However, by 2002, a *New England Journal of Medicine* article reviewing knowledge on IBD described the state of the intestinal flora as a "requisite and perhaps central factor in the development of inflammatory bowel disease." In other words, intestinal flora plays a key role in IBD.

As of this writing, a plethora of articles have been published that begin to describe the complex relationship between intestinal flora and the human immune system. Scientists have a better understanding of:

- how "good bacteria" compete with harmful bacteria for receptors on intestinal cell tissue

- how these bacteria interact with the epithelial cells to regulate the immune response

- how probiotics suppress infectious agents

- how the beneficial bacteria reduce intestinal permeability associated with leaky gut[8]

These recent studies on the relationship between intestinal bacteria and intestinal health show that the underlying rationale for the SCD is correct. However, probiotics alone are only part of the approach of the SCD. The other step, only eating foods that can be properly digested, is just as important.

What Can I Eat on the SCD?

The SCD works by only including foods that an injured intestine can digest, avoiding carbohydrates that continue microbial overgrowth. The SCD includes fresh and frozen vegetables, unprocessed meat and fish, homemade yogurt, fruit, cheeses with low lactose content, cooking and salad oils, honey, eggs, nut flours, nuts, and several types of lentils.

When introducing the diet, it is important to follow the instructions in *Breaking the Vicious Cycle*. When first flipping through the book and reading recipes for the diet, I was suffering from a bad bout of ulcerative colitis. My first thought was, "I can't have raw vegetables. Forget about a salad!" However, the diet is progressive; foods such as raw vegetables are not introduced until symptoms such as diarrhea have subsided. For some foods, even more time is needed for the intestine to heal. Dried legumes, for example, should not be tried for at least three months after beginning the diet.

The first months are the most difficult: gaining a firm understanding of how the diet works, paying more attention to labels, spending more time in the kitchen, and slowly introducing new foods. It is also important to follow the diet 100 percent. In the first months, ingesting *any* amount of illegal ingredients may impede progress. However, these months may also be quite rewarding as digestion improves. As Elaine once noted on an e-mail list, "Better to spend your time in the kitchen than in the bathroom."

The following chart gives an overview of the types food included, and not included, on the diet.

OVERVIEW OF FOODS ON THE SPECIFIC CARBOHYDRATE DIET

	Legal	Illegal	Notes
Meat and Fish	Fresh or frozen: poultry, fish, beef, lamb, and shellfish	Processed meats such as hot dogs, cold cuts, and fast food; Most smoked meats and fish	■ Processed meats and most smoked meats contain sugars and other additives. ■ Some canned fish and cured meats meats may be safe if they contain no sugars, additives, or preservatives.
Vegetables	Most fresh or frozen vegetables, including carrots, broccoli, onions, tomato, squashes, and many others; Canned vegetables	Potatoes, yams, and other starchy root vegetables; Packaged vegetables with additional sugars or preservatives	■ Some dried or pickled vegetables may be safe if they contain no sugars, additives, or preservatives.
Fruit	Fresh or frozen fruit with no added sugar, such as bananas (with ripe, speckled small brown spots), apples, pears, and others; Dried fruit with no added sugars or other preservatives/additives	Canned fruit with added sugars or other additives; Dried fruit with added sugars or other additives	■ Fruit should not be tried while diarrhea is active. ■ When first adding fruit to the diet, peel and cook it.
Grains	Grains are not included on the diet	Grains, including bread, rice, pasta, cereal, and products with corn	■ These grains contain carbohydrates that are not properly digested by an injured intestine. Undigested, they become the primary source of energy for harmful bacteria.
Dairy	Homemade yogurt (see page 19); Natural cheeses where the whey is removed and the remaining lactose is "cured," such as Cheddar, Colby, Havarti, Monterey Jack, Parmesan, Swiss, and others; Dry curd cottage cheese (also known as farmer's cheese or hoop cheese); Butter	Milk; Processed cheese, such as American cheese; Fresh cheeses, such as mozzarella and ricotta; Cheese with additives or coloring; Milk products, such as ice cream; Margarine	■ Homemade yogurt is fermented for a longer amount of time to reduce the lactose content. ■ Check the online resources on page 211 for other allowable cheeses.
Oils	Cooking oils, including those made with grains, such as olive, vegetable, canola, and sesame oil	Cooking oils with additives, such as cooking sprays	

	Legal	Illegal	Notes
Nuts	Nut flours, such as blanched almond flour and pecan flour; Nuts with no additives, such as almonds, Brazil nuts, raw cashews, hazelnuts, pecans, and pine nuts; Nut butters with no additives, especially added sugar, such as cashew butter and peanut butter; Nut extracts with no additives	Nuts with added starches, such as those in nut mixes; Pre-chopped nuts with preservatives; Prechopped nuts with preservatives (e.g., the preservative BHT)	■ Use nuts only in the form of nut flour until diarrhea has cleared up. ■ Be cautious of roasted nuts, especially cashews, which often have unlisted additives (see food labeling information on pages 20-21). ■ Wait six months before trying peanuts. ■ Nut flours, such as almond flour, may be purchased in bulk (see the resources section on page 211 for details). ■ Almond flour and almond butter must be made from blanched almonds.
Legumes/Beans	Dry white beans (also called navy or haricot), lentils, lima beans, split peas, and yellow split peas	Soybeans, bean sprouts, black-eyed beans, fava beans, garbanzo beans, and pinto beans; Canned beans; Bean flour (not soaked prior to grinding)	■ Legumes and beans should not be tried until three months after diarrhea has subsided. ■ Prepare beans and lentils by soaking overnight, 10 to 14 hours. Change the water halfway through the soaking process. Also, rinse the beans at the end of the soaking. ■ By soaking the beans, the starches begin to break down. ■ Check online resources (see page 211) for other allowable beans.
Sweeteners	Honey; Saccharin in small quantities	Starches, and added sugar, including corn syrup, high-fructose corn syrup, cane sugar, and molasses; Maple syrup; Stevia; Chocolate, carob, and cocoa	
Spices	Spices of all kinds (with no added starch or anticaking agents)	Spice mixes (these usually have added ingredients)	■ Buy individual spices, not mixtures. ■ Read the ingredients, because even major brands of salt have added sugar in the form of dextrose.
Drinks	Fruit juices with no added sugars; Very dry wine	Juices packed in boxes; Beer, sherry, cordials, liqueurs, or brandy	When diarrhea is active, do not have orange juice in the morning. Be especially careful when purchasing fruit juices. If you don't seem to tolerate a particular brand, sugars may have been added that are not on the ingredients list.

Making SCD Yogurt

Homemade yogurt is an important aspect of the SCD. Natural acidophilus in the yogurt assists with intestinal healing.

Yogurt fermentation requires a constant temperature between 100°F and 110°F (38°C to 43°C). Although this may be accomplished using the heat of a gas oven or by placing a higher wattage light bulb in an electric oven, it makes more sense to invest in a yogurt maker. Here are the basic instructions for making SCD yogurt with a yogurt maker.

SCD Yogurt

INGREDIENTS

- 2 quarts whole milk (goat's milk may also be used)

- 10 grams Yogourmet yogurt starter*

Pour the milk into a large saucepan and place on a stovetop burner over medium heat. Stir the milk frequently to prevent it from sticking to the sides and bottom of the pan. As soon as the milk begins to simmer, remove it from the heat. Be careful—if the pan is too small, you run the risk of the milk boiling over. (If using goat's milk, be careful not to let the temperature exceed 185°F [85°C].)

Allow the milk to cool to room temperature. Skim off any milk that has solidified on top.

Remove the inner container from the yogurt maker and add one cup (235 ml) of milk from the saucepan to the container. Thoroughly mix in the yogurt starter. Add the remaining cooled milk and mix again.

Fill the outer container of the yogurt maker with warm water to the appropriate mark. Place the inner container back into the yogurt maker, turn it on, and allow the yogurt to ferment for a minimum of 24 hours. (Don't leave it in for more than 34 hours.)

Remove the inner container and refrigerate.

*NOTE: Use the "Yogourmet freeze-dried yogurt starter," not the "Casei Bifidus Acidophilus yogurt starter."

A Note on Probiotics

Probiotics are living organisms that, when ingested, may improve the balance of intestinal microflora. In 2005, probiotic sales in the United States reached $243 million. However, there are many strains of probiotics, not all of which are helpful. If purchasing a probiotic supplement, please keep in mind the following:

1. Ideally, buy a supplement with *Lactobacillus acidophilus (L. acidophilus)* as the only strain. Many brands have additional strains of "good bacteria." *S. thermophilus* and *L. bulgaricus* are okay, but avoid anything with bifidobacteria or bifidus.

   Approximately thirty strains of bifidobacteria have been identified, with names such as *Bifidobacterium breve, Bifidobacterium longum*, and *Bifidobacterium infantis*. Although strains of bifidobacteria are included in many probiotics, based on Elaine Gottschall's experience, these strains have a tendency to overgrow in the large intestine and should not be used.

2. Do not buy product with fructooligosaccharides, or "FOS." It may feed the harmful bacteria that the diet is attempting to deprive of energy.

3. Ask around to make sure the company or brand is reputable.

Reading Labels and "SCD-Safe"

A friend who had recently graduated from journalism school was having trouble sleeping at night. After several weeks and lots of research, he started keeping a food diary and found his insomnia came from something he ate. His comment on the experience: "You need a Ph.D. to use the supermarket!" Labels can be tricky.

Here are some items to be aware of:

1. Added sugars are not always included in the ingredients list. Current labeling laws allow companies to omit ingredients that make up less than 5 percent of a product.[9] This does not include allergens, such as gluten, eggs, and peanuts. However, products may include added sugars without declaring them.

   These laws are spelled out by the CODEX Alimentarius Commission, an organization that defines international food standards. It was started in 1963 as a joint project between the World Health Organization and the Food and Agriculture Organization of the United Nations. Go to www.codexalimentarius.net for more information.

2. Be cautious when buying spices and powders. Until recently, it was difficult to purchase spices without caking agents and other additives. However, more grocery stores (notably Whole Foods) stock brands of spices without any additives. Double-check—even common brands of salt contain sugar.

3. Certain ingredients in this book—bacon, for example—are marked "SCD-safe." This is not a brand name but a note to double-check ingredients to make sure they do not include additives, especially starch or sugar.

On to the Recipes

In the years before starting the SCD, illness (read: diarrhea, cramping, and pain) stopped me from traveling. Many trips, whether away for the weekend, or, in one instance, an invitation to see the Summer Olympics in Barcelona, were cancelled or declined.

However, with the SCD, and some pre-prepared food for longer flights, I have since been on many overseas trips, including six trips to India. I take flights within the United States, whether for work, weddings, or simply to get away, for granted. Thankfully, the SCD has allowed me to see other parts of the world, and it's been many years since an overnight trip seemed like a serious matter.

Similarly, in this book, I have tried to expand the reach of the diet by exploring different world cuisines and adapting dishes for the SCD. I hope you have as much fun making these recipes as I did—washing, chopping, slicing, peeling, grating, mixing, stirring, baking, frying, boiling, steaming, eating, drinking … enjoy!

1. Nieves, R., and R.T. Jackson. "Specific carbohydrate diet in treatment of inflammatory bowel disease." *Tennessee Medicine*, 2004; 97(9): 407.

2. Haas, Sidney, and Merrill P. Haas. *Management of Celiac Disease*. Philadelphia: J.P. Lippincott Company, 1951, pp. 6–8.

3. *New York Times*. "Dr. Sidney Haas Valentine Dies; Pediatrician and Researcher, 94." December 1, 1964.

4. Haas, Sidney. *Management of Celiac Disease*. Philadelphia: J.P. Lippincott Company, 1951, pp. 128–129.

5. *New York Times*. "Banana Shortage Serious; Originator of the Treatment for Celiac Disease Explains Problem"; August 6, 1942, p. 18.

6. Borruel, N., et al. 2002. "Increased mucosal tumour necrosis factor alpha production in Crohn's disease can be downregulated ex vivo by probiotic bacteria." *Gut*; 51:659–664.

7. *Acta Paediatrica*, 2005. "Tight junctions, leaky intestines, and pediatric disease." 94:4 pp. 386–393.

8. *The Journal of Nutrition*, 2007. "Probiotic effects on inflammatory bowel disease." Vol. 137:3, suppl. 2, pp. 819–4S.

9. General Standards for the Labeling of Prepackaged Foods, Codex Stan 1-1985 (Rev. 1-1991).

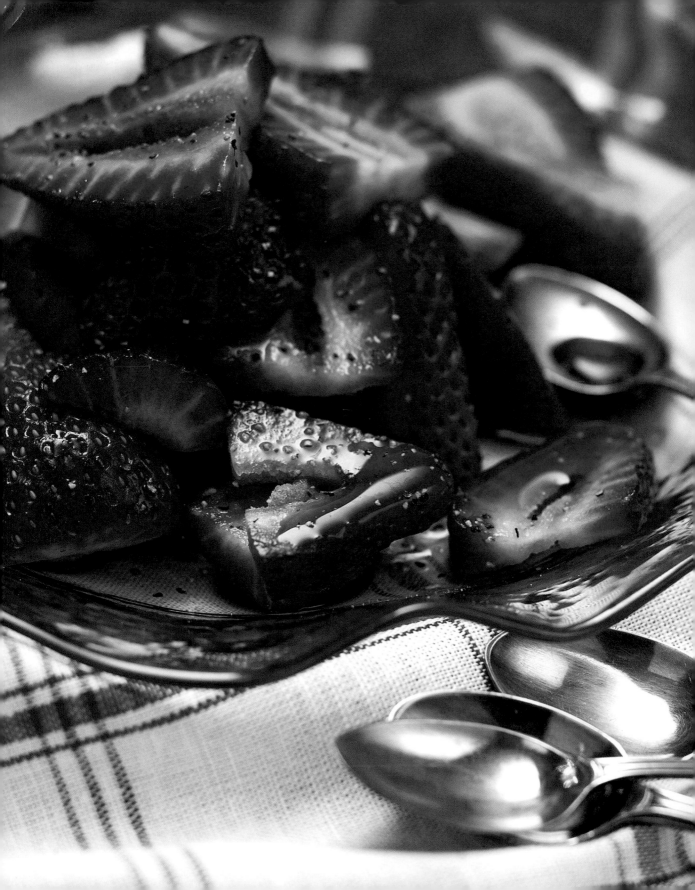

CHAPTER 1

Breakfast

A few years ago, we were introduced to a wonderful New Year's Eve tradition: writing down instances from the previous year—events, thoughts, names of people, or moments that one wants to leave behind—on small slips of paper.

At the stroke of the New Year, you must throw these slips into the fireplace, so as to burn away all those negative instances. Or, in our case, light them in a fire-proof bucket on the back porch in the freezing winter.

Out with the old! Our recent New Year's Eve celebrations have been small, with lots of eating, drinking, and laughing. The half-hour before midnight takes on a more solemn tone when everyone starts writing down events that each would rather forget.

"Hey, put that down! You can't read other people's slips!"

Well, almost solemn. By the time the ball drops, the ashes settle, and everyone falls asleep, there's little energy left. Refueling means a morning with pots of trade coffee;* giant omelets with vegetables, onions, and cheese; and fluffy pancakes.

In my case, the small cast-iron pan is brought out for special SCD hazelnut-vanilla pancakes with a distinctive, delicious crunch. It's a good way—in moderation—to start off the New Year.

*NOTE: Coffee may be introduced when symptoms have settled down. Because of the chemicals, however, decaf should be avoided.

Hazelnut-Vanilla Pancakes

You don't have to stare longingly anymore (especially during wintry morning commutes) at those highway billboards featuring soft, fluffy pancakes. Create your own fluffy version in the warmth of your kitchen—whether it is for a Sunday brunch or a pre-commute indulgence.

INGREDIENTS

PANCAKES

- 1 cup (110 g) almond flour
- 1/4 cup (40 g) hazelnuts
- 4 eggs
- 2 tablespoons (40 g) honey
- 1 teaspoon vanilla extract
- 1/4 teaspoon salt
- 1/4 teaspoon baking soda
- Butter, for frying

VANILLA-INFUSED HONEY SYRUP

- 1/16 teaspoon vanilla extract
- 1/2 cup (170 g) honey
- 1 cinnamon stick (optional)

To make the pancakes, blend together all the ingredients, except the butter, in a food processor.

Butter a pancake griddle or nonstick stovetop pan, and pour the pancake batter in spoonfuls onto the pan. Scoop only enough batter to cover the surface thinly. The thinner you make the pancakes, the more evenly and easily they will cook through.

Fry until golden on the bottom, and then flip and cook until golden on the other side.

To make the syrup, heat all of the syrup ingredients in a pan until combined, approximately 1 minute. Drizzle on top of the pancakes and serve.

YIELD: 3 large or 6 small pancakes

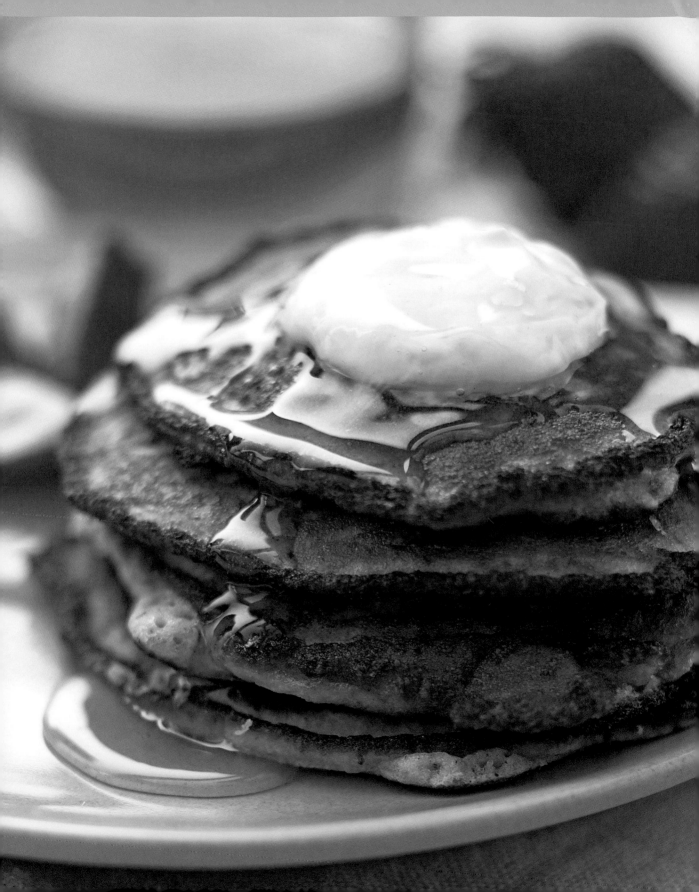

Butternut Squash Hazelnut Muffins

These muffins are great fresh and warm out of the oven, or packed away as a handy snack when you are traveling for the weekend.

INGREDIENTS

- One 1 1/2- to 2-pound (685- to 910-g) butternut squash
- 1/4 cup (55 g) butter, melted
- 3/4 cup (255 g) honey
- 2 eggs
- 1 cup (110 g) almond flour
- 1 cup (145 g) hazelnuts
- 1 teaspoon baking soda
- 1 teaspoon cinnamon powder
- 1/2 teaspoon nutmeg powder
- 1/2 teaspoon ginger powder
- 1/2 teaspoon clove powder

Preheat the oven to 325°F (170°C, or gas mark 3). Cut the butternut squash in half, scoop out the seeds, and steam the halves until soft, approximately 20 minutes. Scoop out the insides of the squash and purée in a food processor. Measure out 1 1/2 cups (340 g) puréed squash.

Butter 2 nonstick muffin tins and set aside. Add the butter, honey, eggs, and 1 1/2 cups (340 g) squash to the food processor and blend. Finally, add the almond flour, hazelnuts, baking soda, cinnamon, nutmeg, ginger, and clove powders, and mix until thoroughly blended.

Spoon the muffin batter into the muffin pans.

Bake until a knife inserted into the center of a muffin comes out clean, approximately 20 minutes.

YIELD: 16 muffins

Mom's Blueberry Muffins

My mother rises early—she likes her morning time to herself—while the rest of the house is still asleep. She takes the dog out for a walk, enjoys her cup of morning coffee, and creates delectable breakfast goodies for us to enjoy. The aroma of fresh blueberry muffins wafting through her warm sunny kitchen greets us when we wake, along with a smile and "good morning."

INGREDIENTS

- 2 ½ cups (275 g) almond flour
- 4 tablespoons (55 g) butter, melted
- 1 teaspoon baking soda
- ¼ teaspoon salt
- ¼ teaspoon nutmeg
- ⅓ cup (115 g) honey
- 1 teaspoon vanilla extract
- ⅓ cup (85 g) SCD Yogurt (page 19)
- 2 eggs
- 1 cup (145 g) fresh blueberries,* plus 24 more for garnish

Preheat the oven to 325°F (170°C, or gas mark 3). Line 2 mini-muffin pans with muffin liners or grease the muffin tins.

Place all the ingredients, except the blueberries, in a food processor and process until well mixed. Fold in the blueberries. Pour the mixture into the muffin pans. Garnish the top of each muffin with a blueberry.

Bake for 15 to 20 minutes, or until a toothpick inserted into a muffin comes out clean.

YIELD: 24 mini-muffins

*NOTE: Wait at least three months after symptoms have cleared before trying blueberries.

Raisin-Raspberry Scones

Scones always bring to mind afternoon high tea in an old manor house situated in the rolling English countryside. But you don't need to hop on a plane to enjoy these homemade, sumptuous treats.

INGREDIENTS

- 5 tablespoons (70 g) butter, melted
- 1/4 cup (62 g) SCD Yogurt (page 19)
- 2 eggs
- 1 teaspoon vanilla extract
- 3/4 teaspoon baking soda
- 1/4 teaspoon salt
- 1/2 teaspoon cardamom powder
- 1/3 cup (115 g) honey
- 1/4 cup (35 g) raisins
- 1/4 cup (30 to 60 g) raspberries,* frozen or fresh
- 2 cups (220 g) almond flour

Preheat the oven to 350°F (180°C, or gas mark 4). Grease a large baking tray.

In a food processor, blend together all the ingredients except the almond flour. Make sure the batter is well puréed. Add the almond flour to the mixture and blend again.

Drop batter onto the greased baking tray, in 2-inch circles that are evenly spaced. Bake for 15 minutes, or until the edges turn golden brown and/or a knife inserted into a scone comes out clean.

YIELD: 10 to 14 scones

*****NOTE:** Wait at least three months after symptoms have cleared before trying raspberries.

Fresh Fruit and Yogurt with Homemade Trail Mix

I usually wake up to find our dog hovering near the bed, ready to go for a morning walk. After a 25-minute loop around the neighborhood, I usually end up at the local coffee shop to get my wife her morning coffee. But the best part of the morning is when I get back home for a "bowl of breakfast," such as the one below.

INGREDIENTS

- ½ apple, peeled and cut into bite-size pieces
- 1 banana, peeled and cut into pieces
- ½ teaspoon honey

- ¼ cup (55 g) Raman's Trail Mix (page 76)
- ¼ cup (112 g) dry curd cottage cheese
- ½ cup (112 g) SCD Yogurt (page 19)

Mix all the ingredients together in a bowl. Enjoy!

YIELD: 1 to 2 servings

NOTE: You can substitute other fruit, such as one small pear, peeled and cut into pieces, or half a mango, peeled and cut into pieces.

Early Morning Smoothie

One morning, I discovered our long-lost blender, and since then I often "drink" my breakfast in the form of a smoothie.

INGREDIENTS

- ½ cup (112 g) dry curd cottage cheese
- ½ cup (112 g) SCD Yogurt (page 19)

- ½ cup (120 ml) SCD-safe apple juice (see chart on pages 17–18)
- 1 banana

Combine all the ingredients together in a blender until smooth. Pour into glass, and enjoy!

YIELD: 1 tall glass

NOTE: You can also add ingredients such as 4 or 5 pecans or one-quarter of an apple or other fruit.

Huevos Rancheros

Snow peas add an unusual crunch to this traditional Mexican breakfast dish. Meaning "eggs country-style" in Spanish. this dish was often served as a late-morning or early afternoon treat for farm laborers working since the crack of dawn.

INGREDIENTS

- 6 eggs
- 1 teaspoon olive oil
- 1 small onion, finely chopped
- 1 Anaheim chile, deseeded and finely chopped
- 9 chives, finely chopped
- 10 snow peas, finely chopped
- 1 medium tomato, finely chopped
- 1/4 teaspoon oregano
- 1/4 cup (15 g) fresh cilantro, finely chopped
- Salt and pepper to taste
- 1/4 to 1/2 ounce (8 to 15 g) grated Gruyère cheese

Break the eggs into a bowl, mix, and set aside.

Heat the olive oil in a nonstick pan over medium heat, and add the onion and Anaheim chile. Sauté and allow the onion and chile to brown, 3 to 4 minutes.

Add the chives and snow peas to the pan, and cook together for about 1 minute. Next, add the chopped tomato and cook until soft, 2 to 4 minutes. Sprinkle the oregano into the mixture, and add the eggs. Throw in the cilantro immediately. Add salt and pepper to taste.

Allow the eggs to cook for 3 to 5 minutes until they reach the desired consistency, stirring often to make sure they do not stick to the pan. Top with the grated cheese.

YIELD: 3 servings (approximately 2 eggs per person)

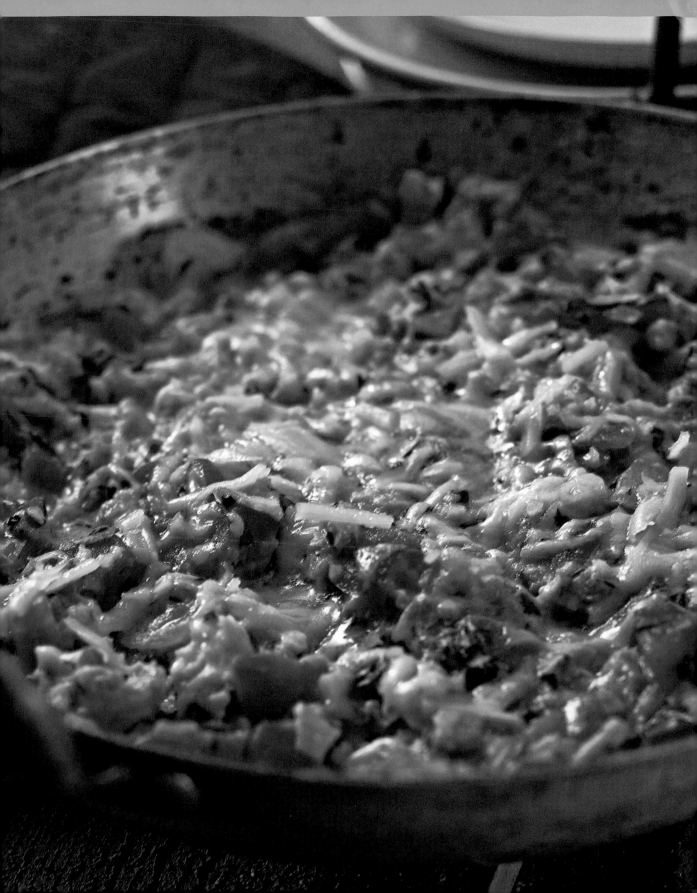

Grandma Joan's Zucchini Omelet

In the midst of working on this recipe book, we went to visit our friends, Frank and Nicole, and their son Augie. We stayed at Augie's grandmother's house during our visit and enjoyed a weekend filled with food, laughter, and mural drawing. Waking up on Sunday, Joan greeted us with a delicious omelet cooked to perfection, all ready and laid out on the dining table.

INGREDIENTS

- 1 onion, thinly sliced
- 1/3 red bell pepper, cored, seeded, and finely chopped
- 3 teaspoons olive oil, divided
- 1 medium or 2 small zucchinis, grated
- 5 eggs
- 1/2 teaspoon salt
- 1/2 teaspoon pepper
- 2 to 4 tablespoons (14 to 28 g) SCD-safe sun-dried tomatoes (see chart on pages 17–18)
- 2 tablespoons (14 g) almond slivers
- 1/2 cup (60 g) Cheddar cheese, grated

In a stovetop pan, sauté the onion and bell pepper in 1 teaspoon of the olive oil for 4 to 5 minutes and set aside.

Heat the remaining 2 teaspoons olive oil over medium heat in a large, non-stick frying pan, preferably one that has a fitted lid. Layer the bottom of the frying pan with grated zucchini. Once it has lightly browned, add the onion and bell pepper and lightly sauté.

Whisk the eggs together in a small bowl. Pour the eggs into the pan. Add the salt, pepper, sun-dried tomatoes, and almond slivers.

Sprinkle the top with the Cheddar cheese so that the omelet is almost completely covered.

Cover the pan with a tight-fitting lid and reduce the heat to low. The omelet will puff slightly when done.

YIELD: 5 to 6 servings

Sara's Omelet

We were visiting a close family friend who had recently moved. We don't have a chance to meet so often anymore, but when we do get together, the omelet she makes stands out in my memory. This omelet comes out light and fluffy because of the dual process of stovetop cooking and oven baking.

INGREDIENTS

- 1 tablespoon (14 g) butter
- 1 tablespoon (15 ml) olive oil
- 1 onion, finely chopped
- 1 red bell pepper, finely chopped
- 10 small mushrooms, finely chopped
- 1 teaspoon oregano
- 8 eggs
- 1 teaspoon water
- Salt and pepper to taste
- 3/4 cup (90 g) grated Gruyère or Cheddar cheese

Preheat the oven to 350°F (180°C, or gas mark 4).

Warm the butter and oil in a stovetop (and ovenproof) pan over medium heat. Add the onion, pepper, and mushrooms. Cook until the mushrooms have given off water and turned brown and the onions have caramelized, 5 to 10 minutes. Add the oregano.

Meanwhile, whisk the eggs with the water. Add the salt and pepper. Add the grated cheese to the eggs.

Reduce the stovetop heat to low, and stir the eggs into the mixture. Once the eggs begin to set, transfer the pan to the oven and cook until the eggs set, 10 to 15 minutes.

YIELD: 6 servings

Bacon Eggs Benedict

This is a perfect Sunday morning brunch—especially if you make it for someone as a surprise.

INGREDIENTS

- 3 strips SCD-safe bacon (see chart on pages 17–18)
- 1 teaspoon olive oil
- 2 scallions, halved and then cut vertically into thin strips
- 2 eggs
- 1 square Olive Sandwich Bread (page 41)
- 2 to 3 tablespoons (30 to 45 g) Angie's Hollandaise Sauce (page 171)
- Salt and pepper to taste

Cook the bacon strips in a small pan on the stovetop and set aside.

Heat the olive oil over medium heat in a nonstick pan, and cook the scallions in the olive oil for about 1 minute. Add the eggs. Allow them to cook to the desired consistency. (Eggs Benedict usually have slightly soft yolks, but if you prefer, you can cook them until firm.)

On a plate, place the bread as the base layer and then add the bacon. Top this with the cooked eggs and then dribble over with the Hollandaise sauce. Add salt and pepper to taste.

YIELD: 1 serving

NOTE: The flavor comes from the combination of bread, egg, and Hollandaise sauce.

CHAPTER 2

Savory Baked Goods

As small children, my sister and I were sometimes sequestered inside rooms while our parents played pinochle with their friends. One night we took out paper and crayons with the goal of constructing dream sandwiches, impossible stacks of cheese slices, tomato, chicken, lettuce, hamburger, onion, pickles, ketchup, peanut butter, bananas, mayo, mustard … everything all at once. (Everything that tasted good separately, but not necessarily together.)

In later weeks, we attempted actual construction of these sandwiches. We never stacked even half the ingredients before the towers of food slid over and collapsed—even half-size towers were too much for us to fit into our mouths.

Some of these experiments must have stuck in my memory. Every few weeks, as a late afternoon break, I attempt mini-sandwiches. Thinly sliced almond flour bread. Simple combinations. Peanut butter and banana. Avocado and tomato. Melted cheese and chicken. Whatever is within reach …

Cilantro-Onion Sticks

These "breadsticks" are great on their own, or with the Cilantro Dip/Spread (page 179).

INGREDIENTS

- 3 egg whites
- 2 cloves garlic, grated
- $^1/_3$ cup (55 g) finely chopped onion
- $^1/_4$ teaspoon salt
- $^1/_4$ teaspoon black pepper
- $^1/_8$ teaspoon baking soda
- 2 tablespoons (8 g) finely chopped fresh cilantro
- 2 to 2 $^1/_2$ cups (220 to 275 g) almond flour

Preheat the oven to 350°F (180°C, or gas mark 4). Grease a baking tray (you can grease with oil to make sure this is a dairy-free recipe).

In a medium-size bowl, beat the egg whites until stiff. Set aside.

In a separate bowl, mix together the garlic, onion, salt, pepper, baking powder, fresh cilantro, and almond flour.

Slowly fold in the egg whites. The dough should be moist, but not sticky.

Form $^1/_2$-inch (6-mm) dough balls and roll them between your palms to make long strands (sticks). Gently place the rolled sticks on the baking tray well spaced apart. Place in the oven, and bake until the sticks turn golden brown, 20 to 30 minutes.

YIELD: 30 to 35 sticks, depending on the length

NOTE: Instead of sticks, you can make these as regular crackers, by pressing the $^1/_4$-inch (6-mm) dough balls flat onto the baking tray, rather than making them into long strands.

Nilou's Chile-Lime Crackers

My wife secretly stores stashes of these tangy crackers in different jars through-out our kitchen, so that I do not eat them all when they come out of the oven.

INGREDIENTS

- 2 cups grated (230 g) Monterey Jack cheese
- 1 ½ cups (165 g) almond flour
- 3 tablespoons (45 ml) cold water
- ¼ cup (60 ml) olive oil
- ¼ teaspoon minced garlic
- ¼ teaspoon salt
- ⅛ teaspoon turmeric powder
- ¼ teaspoon chili powder
- ¼ teaspoon chile pepper powder
- ¼ teaspoon lime zest
- 2 teaspoons lime juice

Preheat the oven to 350°F (180°C, or gas mark 4). Grease a baking tray.

Mix the ingredients together in a bowl. Form into a ball and refrigerate until firm, about 15 minutes.

Drop small rounds of the dough, well spaced apart, onto the baking tray. Press the dough rounds and flatten onto the tray. Place in the oven, and bake for approximately 15 minutes, or until the crackers turn golden brown.

Allow to cool.

YIELD: 25 to 30 crackers

Curry Crackers

This cracker is packed with lots of good South Asian spiciness. The secret to this recipe is in the Curry Powder (page 175) that we make from original whole spices. This gives the crackers a fresh and pungent flavor. Try it with the Cilantro Dip/Spread (page 179).

INGREDIENTS

- 3 egg whites
- 3 cloves garlic, grated
- 1 spring onion, finely chopped
- ¼ teaspoon cayenne pepper flakes
- ¼ teaspoon salt
- ¼ teaspoon baking powder
- 1 teaspoon Curry Powder (page 175)
- ½ cup (100 g) Parmesan cheese
- 2 to 2 ½ cups (220 to 275 g) almond flour

Preheat the oven to 350°F (180°C, or gas mark 4). Grease a baking tray.

In a medium-size bowl, beat the egg whites until stiff, about 5 minutes. Set aside.

In a separate bowl, mix together the garlic, spring onion, cayenne pepper, salt, baking powder, curry powder, cheese, and almond flour, until thoroughly blended. Slowly fold in the egg whites.

On the greased baking tray, drop small rounds of the batter, well spaced apart. Press the dough rounds and flatten onto the tray. Place in the oven, and bake until the crackers turn golden brown, approximately 15 to 20 minutes, or until a knife inserted into a cracker comes out clean.

YIELD: 25 crackers

NOTE: Additional curry powder may be sprinkled on top.

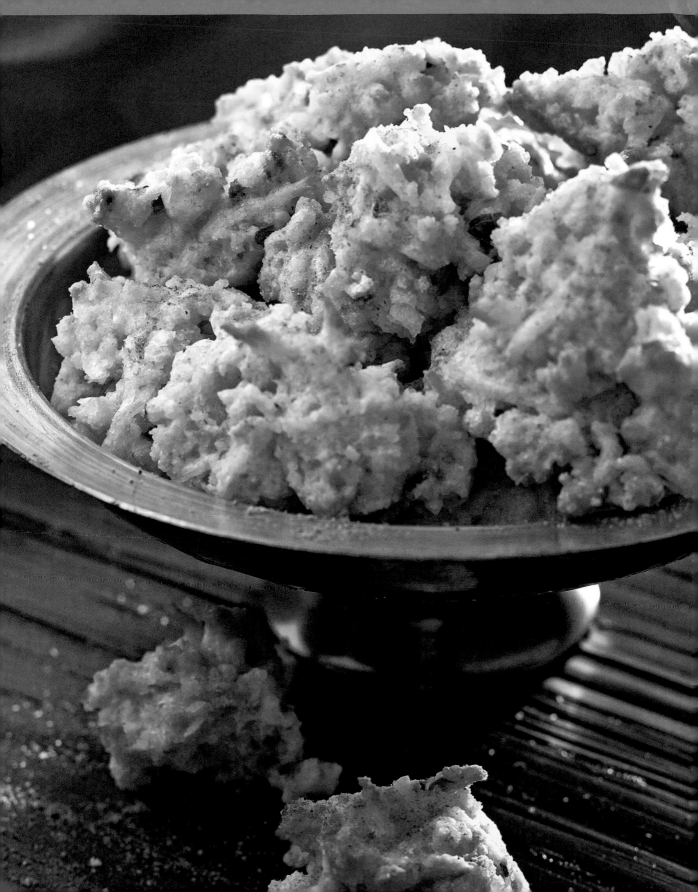

Spicy Herbed Cheese Crackers

The herb mix takes a simple cheese cracker recipe and turns it upside down. The addition of a concentrated coating of herbs is incredibly tasty and delicious. You can serve it with one of the Herb Dips (page 83).

INGREDIENTS
CRACKERS

- 5 ounces (140 g) Cheddar cheese, grated
- 1 cup (110 g) almond flour
- ¼ cup (60 ml) olive oil
- 3 tablespoons (45 ml) water
- ½ teaspoon coarse salt
- ⅛ teaspoon dried dill flakes
- 3 cloves garlic, peeled and minced

HERB MIX

- 1 ¼ teaspoons dried oregano
- 1 ¼ teaspoons dried dill
- 1 teaspoon sea salt

Preheat the oven to 350°F (180°C, or gas mark 4). Grease a baking tray.

To make the crackers, in a mixing bowl, combine the cracker ingredients. The mixture should form a moist but firm dough.

To make the herb mix, combine the ingredients in a small bowl. Make small dough balls, roll them in the herb mix, and flatten on the greased baking tray at even intervals.

Bake for 15 to 20 minutes, until the crackers are golden brown.

YIELD: 30 to 35 crackers, depending on size

NOTE: You can use other herbs for the herb mix, such as oregano and thyme.

Olive Sandwich Bread

The olive loaf has roots in Italy and other parts of the Mediterranean. We created a version for the SCD that is layered with olives, shallots, cheese, and thyme.

INGREDIENTS

- 3 eggs
- 1/2 cup (50 g) finely chopped shallots
- 10 kalamata olives, pitted and finely chopped
- 7 1/2 ounces (210 g) dry curd cottage cheese
- 2 tablespoons (28 g) butter, melted
- 3 tablespoons (15 g) grated Parmesan cheese
- 1/2 teaspoon salt
- 1/2 teaspoon baking soda
- 1/4 teaspoon thyme
- 1/2 cup (125 g) SCD Yogurt (page 19)
- 3 cups (330 g) almond flour
- 2 kalamata olives, pitted and halved, for garnish (optional)

Preheat the oven to 350°F (180°C, or gas mark 4).

Blend together all the ingredients in a food processor until well mixed, 3 to 5 minutes.

Pour into a greased 9- by 13-inch (23- by 33-cm) baking dish. If you like, you can top the bread with evenly spaced olives. Bake in the oven until a knife inserted into the center comes out clean, 30 to 45 minutes.

YIELD: 20 to 25 slices

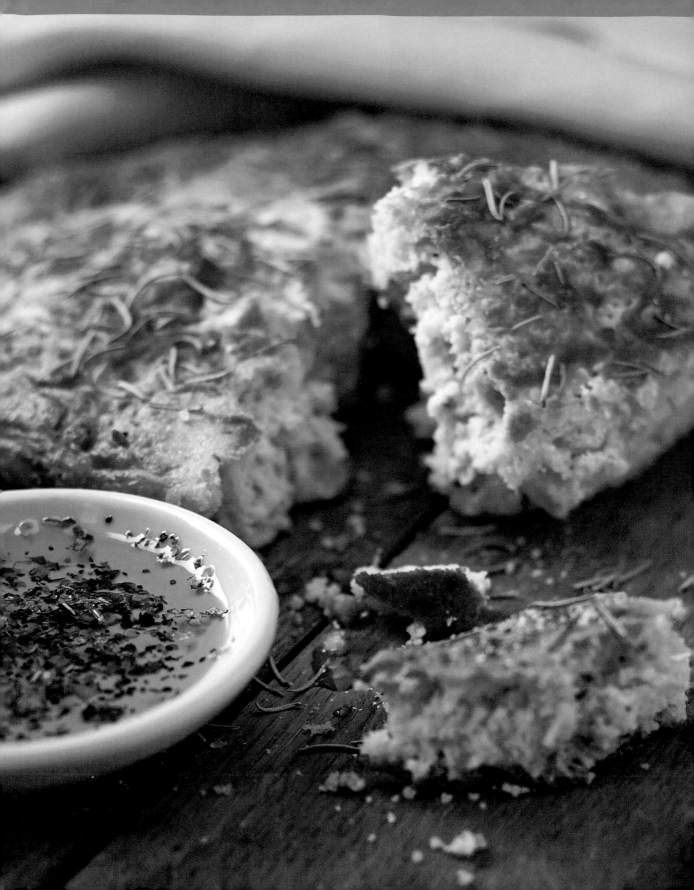

Focaccia

Focaccia has been around since the time of the ancient Greeks, but today, it is well known as a specialty from Genoa, Italy. The focaccia from that area is made with cheese, much as we make it in our recipe below. We use the traditional rosemary topping, but you can improvise with whatever herbs you fancy. Focaccia is great as a sandwich bread for lunch, as a dipping bread, as an appetizer, or as an afternoon snack purely on its own.

INGREDIENTS

BREAD

- 2 cups (220 g) almond flour
- 7 ounces (200 g) dry curd cottage cheese
- 1 teaspoon baking soda
- ¼ teaspoon salt
- ½ teaspoon coarse black pepper
- ½ cup (60 g) grated Cheddar cheese
- 3 eggs
- 3 tablespoons (40 g) butter, melted
- 2 scallion sprigs, finely sliced

TOPPING

- ½ teaspoon coarse sea salt
- 1 tablespoon (8 g) finely grated Cheddar cheese
- 1 teaspoon dried rosemary

Preheat the oven to 375°F (190°C, or gas mark 5). Grease a 9- by 13-inch (23- by 33-cm) baking dish.

To make the bread, mix together the bread ingredients in a food processor until well blended. Remove from the blender and spread out in the greased baking dish.

To make the topping, combine the topping ingredients and mix well. Sprinkle the topping on the bread.

Place in the oven and bake until the edges brown, 30 to 40 minutes.

Allow to cool and then cut into sandwich squares.

YIELD: Approximately 20 squares, depending on size

Sun-Dried Tomato Bread

This Mediterranean-inspired SCD bread is flavored with sun-dried tomatoes and chives.

INGREDIENTS

- 2 eggs
- 1 cup SCD Yogurt (page 19)
- 2 tablespoons (28 g) butter, melted
- 1 teaspoon salt
- 1 teaspoon baking soda
- 1/2 teaspoon pepper
- 3 1/2 cups (385 g) almond flour
- 1/4 cup (12 g) finely chopped chives
- 1/4 cup (14 g) finely chopped sun-dried tomatoes, SCD-safe (see chart on pages 17–18)

Preheat the oven to 325°F (170°C, or gas mark 3). Grease a 9- by 13-inch (23- by 33-cm) baking dish.

Blend together all the ingredients in a food processor. Pour into the greased baking dish.

Bake in the oven for 30 to 40 minutes, until a knife inserted into the center comes out clean.

YIELD: 20 to 25 slices

CHAPTER 3

Soups

When she was a girl, my grandmother used to make soup by first visiting the open-air markets in New Haven, Connecticut. She made her rounds, gathering vegetables: a few carrots from one vendor, some string beans from another. Back home, she'd roast the top of a chuck bone in the oven, then combine the bone and all of the vegetables to make a nutritious soup.

That all sounds well and good, but an interstate highway now runs through New Haven where the open-air markets once flourished, and, after a long workday, hunger's call may be overwhelming. Who has time to make soup?

When I brought this up with my grandmother, Nonnie (as we call her) advised using a Crock-Pot. The Crock-Pot, or slow cooker, is a large ceramic bowl that cooks food over a period of two to ten hours, depending on the recipe and the heat setting. You can turn it on in the morning and have hot food ready when you return from work. In addition, it makes large quantities of food. You can easily make six to eight servings. With the Crock-Pot, there's no excuse not to make soups—or anything else for that matter.

When my grandmother gave me a Crock-Pot many years ago, months went by before I took it out of the box. But I did, after firm words from Nonnie: "If I can use the VCR, you can certainly learn to use the Crock-Pot—it has only one switch!"

This year, my grandmother turned ninety—and she is still cooking away.

Basic Vegetable Soup/Stock

This simple vegetable soup is a great alternative to store-bought soup stocks, which often have preservatives and other SCD-illegal ingredients added to them. We have used dried herbs in this recipe, but you can add fresh ones depending on the season. You could also try other vegetables, such as string beans, cabbage leaves, cauliflower, etc.

INGREDIENTS

- 2 tablespoons (30 ml) olive oil
- 4 cloves garlic, peeled and minced
- 1 large white onion, finely chopped
- 1 large leek, washed, ends trimmed, and finely chopped
- 2 cups (260 g) peeled and finely chopped carrots
- 2 cups (200 g) finely chopped celery
- 2 cups (240 g) finely chopped zucchini
- 2 cups (140 g) finely chopped mushrooms

- 1 large tomato, finely chopped
- 3 bay leaves
- 1 ½ teaspoons salt
- 1 teaspoon black pepper
- 1 teaspoon dried oregano
- 1 teaspoon dried thyme
- 10 cups (2350 ml) water
- Salt and pepper to taste

Heat the olive oil in a large pot and sauté the garlic, onion, and leek over medium heat for 3 to 5 minutes. Add the carrots, celery, zucchini, mushrooms, tomato, bay leaves, salt, pepper, oregano, and thyme and stir-fry for 1 to 2 minutes.

Add the 10 cups of water, increase the heat to high, and bring to a boil. This will take approximately 10 minutes. Reduce the heat to a low simmer, cover the soup pot, and cook for 1 hour.

Remove from the heat and cool.

To make the stock, strain out the vegetables and herbs through a sieve. The resulting strained stock will be clear broth (use this in the recipes where vegetable stock is called for). Discard the vegetable pulp.

YIELD: 10 cups (2350 ml)

Basic Chicken Soup/Stock

This is a basic recipe for chicken soup that we have used for more than ten years. You may throw in additional or different vegetables or herbs, but the great taste comes from simmering everything together for a couple of hours. It is a wholesome soup that will lift your spirits when you are feeling a bit under the weather.

INGREDIENTS

- 1 tablespoon (15 ml) olive oil
- 4 cloves garlic, peeled and minced
- 2 small onions, finely chopped
- 6 carrots, peeled and sliced into rounds
- 3 stalks celery, sliced into rounds
- 2 medium-size zucchini, finely chopped
- 1 sprig fresh rosemary
- 10 fresh sage leaves
- 5 sprigs fresh thyme
- 1 whole chicken, skinned
- 10 cups (2350 ml) water (or enough to cover the chicken in the pot)
- Salt and pepper to taste

Heat the olive oil in a large soup pot and sauté the garlic and onions until slightly browned. Add the carrots, celery, and zucchini, and sauté for 5 to 7 minutes, stirring constantly. Add the rosemary, sage, and thyme, and continue to stir for a few minutes, dispersing the flavors of the herbs.

Drop in the whole chicken, and pour in the water (enough to cover the chicken completely). Add salt and pepper to taste. Bring to a boil, reduce to a simmer, cover, and cook 1 to 1 ½ hours, or until the chicken is done. Remove the chicken bones from the soup before serving.

To make stock, strain the vegetables, herbs, and chicken through a sieve. The resulting strained soup will be clear broth (use this in recipes where chicken stock is called for).

YIELD: 16 cups (3760 ml)

Caribbean Avocado Soup

The avocado and yogurt blend together to create a creamy-textured soup. The curry powder adds a bit of zing and complements the tanginess of the spices. The soup is filling and can be served for lunch or as a light dinner entrée with Focaccia (page 43).

INGREDIENTS

- 3 ripe avocados
- 2 ½ cups (590 ml) Basic Chicken Stock (page 47), divided
- 1 teaspoon Curry Powder (page 175)
- 1 teaspoon salt
- ¼ teaspoon white pepper
- ½ cup (125 g) SCD Yogurt (page 19)

Cut the avocados in half lengthwise, set aside half of an avocado to use for garnish, and scoop out the insides of the remaining 5 halves. Place the avocado flesh into a blender with 1 ½ cups (350 ml) of the chicken stock. Blend.

Add the curry powder, salt, white pepper, yogurt, and remaining 1 cup (240 ml) of stock to the blender. Mix thoroughly. Chill in the refrigerator for 5 to 10 minutes.

To serve, garnish each soup bowl with a few slices of the reserved avocado.

YIELD: 3 ½ cups (825 ml)

NOTE: This recipe must be served immediately. If you leave it too long, the avocado will start turning brown at room temperature and sour.

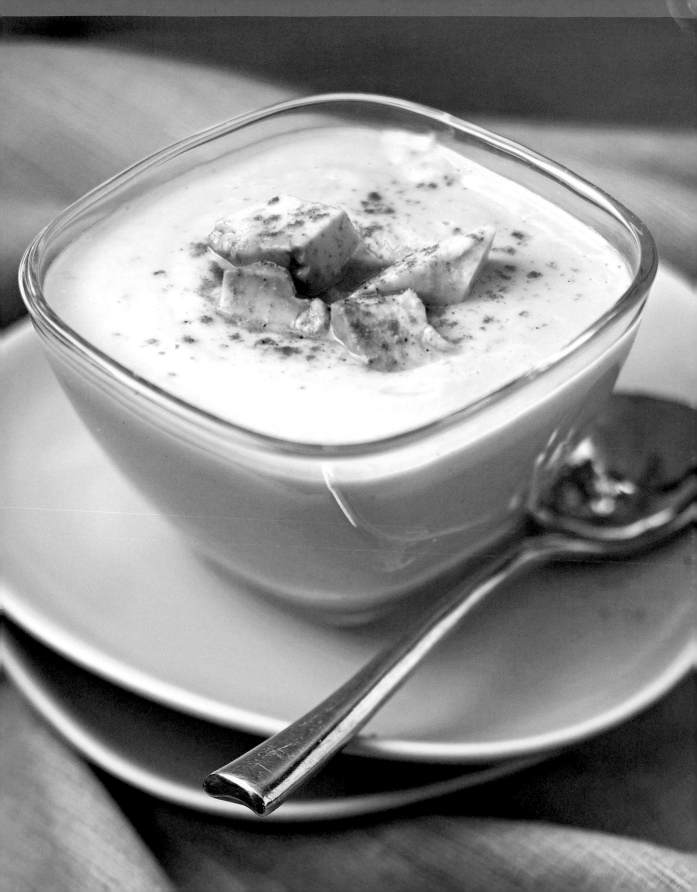

Chandra's Borscht Soup

My younger sister, Chandra, settled down a few years ago. Her husband grew up in Ukraine, so when I asked her for a recipe, the most obvious one was this delicious, nourishing soup, which has its roots in that country. The most incredible part of this soup is the color—a rich, deep maroon.

INGREDIENTS

- 1 large beet
- 1 lime, juiced
- 2 tablespoons (30 ml) olive oil
- 4 cloves garlic, peeled and minced
- 1 red onion, peeled and finely chopped
- 2 bay leaves
- 1 tablespoon salt
- 1/2 tablespoon pepper
- 2 tablespoons (8 g) finely chopped fresh parsley
- 1 large carrot, peeled and finely chopped
- 1 bell pepper, cored, seeded, and finely chopped
- 1/2 cup (35 g) shredded green cabbage
- 2 medium-size celeriac, peeled and cut into small pieces
- 2 medium-size tomatoes, chopped
- 5 or 6 SCD-safe dried apricots, chopped (see chart on pages 17–18)
- 1 1/2 pounds (685 g) beef chuck steak, cubed into small pieces
- 8 cups (1880 ml) Basic Vegetable Stock (page 46)
- 2 cups (470 ml) water

Preheat the oven to 350°F (180°C, or gas mark 4). Wash and dry the beet, and wrap in aluminum foil.

Bake the beet until tender, approximately 30 minutes. Remove from the oven, and allow to cool. Then peel it, cut into small pieces, sprinkle with lime juice, and set aside.

In a large stovetop pot (enough to hold all the soup ingredients), heat the olive oil and add the garlic and onion; cook over medium heat until they turn golden brown. Stir in the bay leaves, salt, pepper, and parsley. Add the carrot, bell pepper, cabbage, celeriac, tomatoes, apricots, and beef. Sauté everything together for 7 to 10 minutes. Pour in the stock and water. Add the oven-roasted beet.

Cover the pot and leave on medium-low heat, until the beef is cooked through and the vegetables are softened, approximately 1 hour.

YIELD: 15 to 16 cups (3525 to 3760 ml)

NOTE: Celeriac is also known as celery root.

Egg Drop Soup

Originating from China, this soup can now be found around the globe, and is so easy to make. All you need are eggs, stock, and water. We have spruced up the basic recipe to provide you with a bit of bite (chives) and additional creaminess (cheese).

INGREDIENTS

- 1/2 cup (50 g) Parmesan cheese, grated
- 1 tablespoon (15 ml) water
- 2 eggs, divided
- 1/2 teaspoon olive oil
- 8 chives
- 4 cups (940 ml) Basic Chicken Stock (page 47)

Whisk together the Parmesan cheese, water, and 1 of the eggs in a small bowl. Set aside. Heat the olive oil in a soup pan and sauté the chives over medium heat for 1 to 2 minutes. Add the stock, bring to a boil, and reduce to a simmer. Stir the reserved egg-drop mixture into the simmering chicken stock. Next, whisk the second egg and then slowly drop it into the soup, stirring slowly for another minute.

Remove from the heat and serve.

YIELD: 4 cups (940 ml)

Leek Soup, Scarborough Fair–style

This soup has a strong seasoning with the rosemary and thyme. After we tasted it, it reminded us of one of our favorite Simon and Garfunkel songs, thus the name.

INGREDIENTS

- 3 large leeks
- 3 tablespoons (42 g) butter
- 1/2 teaspoon crumbled rosemary
- 1 teaspoon thyme
- 1 teaspoon salt, or to taste
- Ground pepper to taste
- 5 cups (1175 ml) Basic Vegetable or Chicken Stock (page 46 or 47)

Wash, trim the edges, and slice the leeks into small pieces. Melt the butter in a soup pot and add the leeks, rosemary, thyme, salt, and pepper. Cook on low heat (do not brown) for approximately 5 minutes. Cover if necessary. When the leeks are tender, add the stock. Bring to a boil, reduce the heat, and simmer for 10 to 15 minutes.

YIELD: 6 cups (1410 ml)

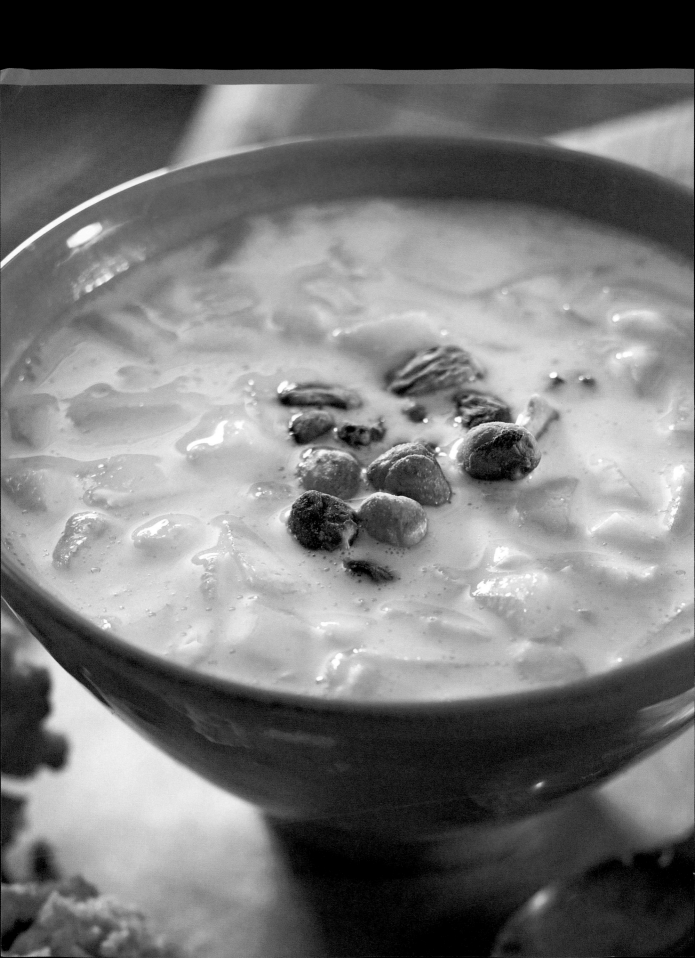

Israeli Tarato Yogurt Soup

This soup has traveled from Spain and Portugal to Bulgaria and finally settled down in Israel. It is made frequently during the hot summer months in that country.

INGREDIENTS

- 2 cups (490 g) SCD Yogurt (page 19)
- 2 cups (470 ml) water
- 1 ¼ tablespoons (20 ml) olive oil
- ½ tablespoon red wine vinegar
- ½ teaspoon salt
- 1 large cucumber
- ½ tablespoon butter
- 15 pistachio nuts, shelled
- 15 shelled peanuts, raw and unsalted

In a large soup pot, combine the yogurt, water, olive oil, vinegar, and salt. Mix together to make sure that the yogurt is well blended into the water and not lumpy. Set aside.

Meanwhile, peel the cucumber, and dice it into small pieces. Add to the soup pot. Alternatively, you could grate the cucumber if you want a different consistency in the soup. If grating, squeeze the excess water out of the cucumber before adding it to the soup. Chill soup in the refrigerator for 1 to 2 hours.

Just before serving, melt the butter in a small sauté pan and add the pistachios and peanuts. Sauté them over medium heat for 1 minute, or until golden brown. Be careful not to burn the nuts. Stir them into the soup.

YIELD: 4 to 5 servings

NOTE: A visiting Israeli friend suggested adding chopped parsley and dill to this soup.

Kenyan Green Pea Soup

When most of us think of East Africa, we visualize going on a safari through wild, untouched spaces. In truth, we are as much an anomaly (and on display) to the animals and birds we seek as they are to us. The globalization of the tourist industry often plays havoc with a specific country's local cuisine, and we had to do a lengthy search to find this delicious soup.

INGREDIENTS

- 1 tablespoon (15 ml) olive oil
- 3 small onions, finely chopped
- 5 cloves garlic, minced
- 1 teaspoon peeled and grated fresh ginger
- 1 teaspoon salt
- 1/4 teaspoon cayenne pepper
- 1/2 teaspoon coriander powder
- 1/2 teaspoon cumin powder
- 2 tomatoes, chopped
- 4 1/2 cups (1060 ml) Basic Vegetable Stock (page 46), divided
- 5 1/2 cups (715 g) frozen green peas

In a soup pot, over medium heat, heat the olive oil and sauté the onions and garlic until they brown. Add the ginger, salt, cayenne, coriander, and cumin powders and cook a few minutes more, stirring often.

Add the tomatoes, and 1 1/2 cups (350 ml) of the vegetable stock. Continue to stir for another 3 to 5 minutes. Turn the heat to high, and bring the soup to a boil. Reduce the heat, cover, and simmer for 5 to 7 minutes. Add the peas and the remaining 3 cups (705 ml) vegetable stock, re-cover the pot, and simmer for 10 to 15 minutes.

Remove from the stovetop, and purée the soup in a blender until smooth.

Serve immediately.

YIELD: 6 cups (1410 ml)

NOTE: This is a dairy-free recipe, but a dollop of SCD Yogurt (see page 19) would give it a delicious creamy texture.

Asparagus Soup

The consistency of this soup is incredibly smooth. In addition to tasting good, asparagus is a vegetable noted for its high level of folic acid—a B-complex vitamin that is often deficient in those with intestinal diseases.

INGREDIENTS

- 2 pounds (910 g) asparagus
- 1 tablespoon (15 ml) olive oil
- 8 spring onions, finely chopped
- 5 cloves garlic
- 1 3/4 pints (830 ml) Basic Vegetable Stock (page 46)
- 1 tablespoon (14 g) butter
- 1/4 teaspoon salt
- 1/4 teaspoon pepper

Clean and prepare the asparagus by cutting and discarding the tough white ends of the stalks. Chop the rest of the asparagus into 1 1/2-inch (3.8-cm) lengths.

Heat the oil in a large saucepan and cook the spring onions and garlic until soft but not browned. Stir in the asparagus, cover the pot, and let the asparagus sweat for 10 minutes. At this stage, remove 5 or 6 asparagus tips to garnish the soup with.

Add the stock, butter, salt, and pepper, and bring to a boil. Stir occasionally. Reduce the heat and let the soup simmer for 25 to 30 minutes, partially uncovered.

In a blender, food processor, or using a hand-held immersion blender, blend the soup in batches until smooth.

Pour the soup into bowls and garnish with the reserved asparagus tips.

YIELD: 5 to 5 1/2 cups (1175 to 1300 ml)

NOTE: Top each serving with a scoop of SCD Yogurt (page 19).

Red Pepper and Tomato Soup

My mother-in-law sent this soup to us with the following instructions: "This soup can be served cold on a hot summer's day, or hot on a cold winter's day." This wonderful, all-season soup is a rich orange-red in color and visually appealing when served in complementary colored bright bowls.

INGREDIENTS

- 2 red peppers
- 7 Roma tomatoes
- 1 tablespoon (15 ml) olive oil
- 1 red onion, thinly sliced
- 1 teaspoon salt
- 1 cup (235 ml) Basic Chicken Stock (page 47)

Preheat the oven to broil. Lightly oil a baking sheet. Bring a pot of water to a boil.

Cut each red pepper into four sections and deseed them. Place them on the lightly oiled baking sheet and broil until the skin starts to wrinkle, 10 to 15 minutes. Turn them over and roast for 5 more minutes. Chop into large pieces and set aside.

Remove the tomato skins by dipping the tomatoes into the pot of boiling water for 30 to 40 seconds. Remove the tomatoes from the pot and dip them into cold water. The peels will slip off. Chop the tomatoes into large pieces. Set aside.

Heat the olive oil over medium heat. Sauté the onion in the oil until golden, 3 to 5 minutes. Place the red pepper, tomatoes, onion, and salt in a food processor and blend to a smooth consistency. Pass through a sieve. Pour the strained mixture into a pot.

Add the chicken stock to the tomato-pepper mixture and bring to a boil. Lower the heat and simmer for 5 minutes. Serve.

YIELD: 3 cups (705 ml)

NOTE: Sprinkle grated cheese over the soup before serving. For this recipe, you would need approximately ½ cup (35 g) grated cheese.

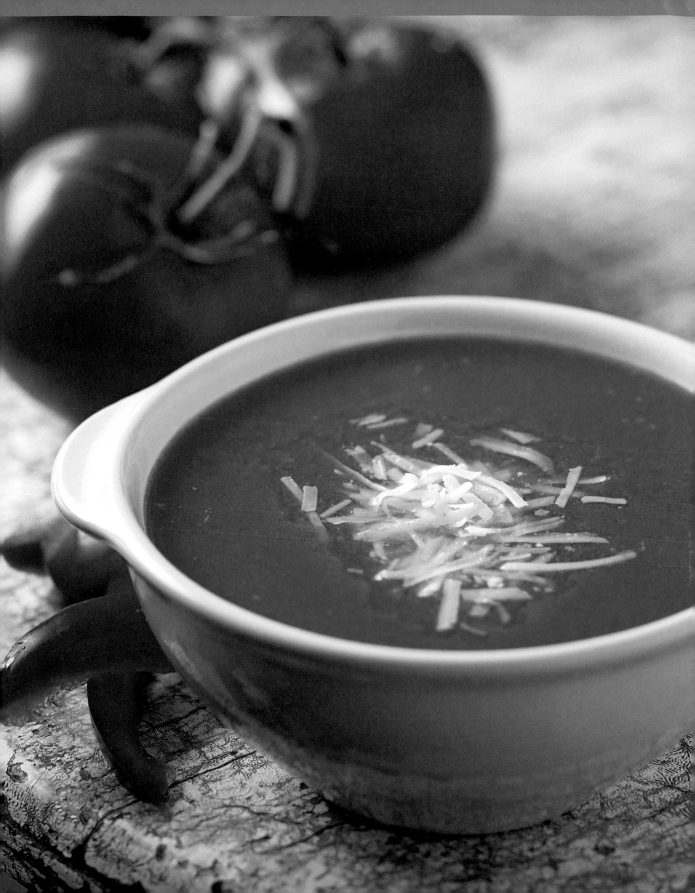

Sophie's Spinach Soup

This soup was sent to us by my older sister-in-law, Sophie. We served this dark green soup at a recent dinner with my younger sister-in-law, Zenobia, and her husband Chris. She enjoyed it so much that she insisted on taking home the leftover soup!

INGREDIENTS

- 1 tablespoon (15 ml) extra virgin olive oil
- 2 medium-size onions, peeled and finely chopped
- 2 cloves garlic, finely minced
- 2 Serrano chiles, seeded and finely chopped
- 1 lemongrass stalk, cut lengthwise
- 1 pound (455 g) fresh spinach, washed and chopped
- 1 cup (235 ml) SCD Coconut Milk* (page 177)
- 2 cups (470 ml) Basic Vegetable Stock (page 46)
- ¼ teaspoon salt
- ¼ teaspoon pepper
- 1 teaspoon unsweetened coconut, finely shredded (optional)

Heat the oil in a deep soup pot and sauté the onions, garlic, and chiles with the lemongrass pieces over medium heat, stirring occasionally, for 3 to 5 minutes. Add the spinach and cook until it starts to wilt, 2 to 4 minutes. Add the coconut milk, stock, salt, and pepper, and bring the soup to a boil. Reduce the heat and simmer for 10 to 15 minutes.

Remove from the stovetop and allow the soup to cool. Remove the lemongrass stalks. Purée the mixture in a food processor or blender until smooth.

When serving, garnish the soup with toasted coconut, if desired. To do this, dry-roast (without oil) the shredded coconut in a small pan on the stovetop until slightly browned.

YIELD: 5 cups (1175 ml)

*****NOTE:** Coconut milk may be tried after six months on the diet.

CHAPTER 4

Salads

Ieat salads often, at least three times a week. Pre-washed. Triple-washed. Organic. Bagged. Loose leaf. Direct from the farm. Iceberg, romaine, crisp head, red leaf, hydroponically grown, butterhead, Boston, Bibb, arugula, garden rocket, and spinach leaves.

However, it's only a few times a year that I get to eat my favorite leaves—when my mother's garden is ready and I happen to visit. Growing up, my siblings and I never paid much attention to her backyard work. (My father did his best to stay away, lest he get caught and end up spending the day tilling or spreading hay.)

Now we understand why her vegetables taste so good. Thirty years ago, she stopped using any type of pesticide and opted for manure and hay instead of chemical fertilizers. For the same amount of time, she has been composting, steadily building up the soil. Some garden debris, including excess brush from tearing out stems and branches, is strategically arranged along the garden fence lines. These areas become sheltering places for song sparrows and swamp sparrows, both of which nest on the ground and like to eat bugs.

These and other natural strategies make her vegetable garden an ecological haven in the middle of the suburbs. During spring and summer, she grows tomatoes, eggplant, zucchini, butternut squash, acorn squash, snap peas, carrots, onions, garlic, beets, pumpkins, and, of course, lettuce leaves. Once the lettuce is ready, she washes, cuts, and places it on a plate with a little oil and vinegar, ready to eat.

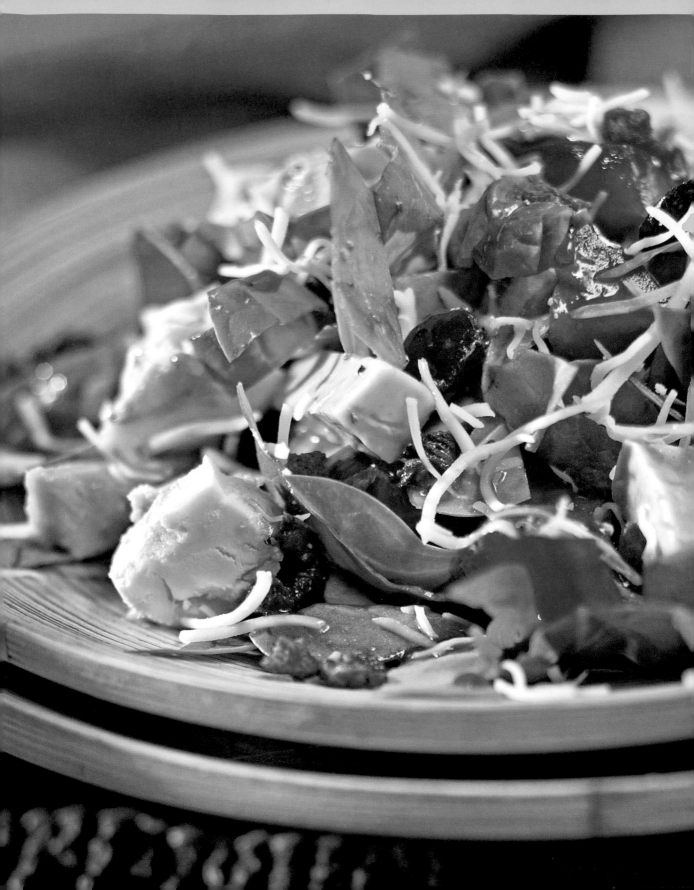

Cobb Salad with Angie's Vinaigrette

When I was still new to the SCD diet and had moved to New York, I worried about finding places to eat. As I eased into life in the city, I found that it was simple to request modifications at most restaurants. However, there was one dish at Time Cafe near Astor Place that did not require any substitutions—an excellent Cobb salad. Below is an attempt to recreate it, and we paired it with a vinaigrette recipe a friend gave us.

INGREDIENTS

SALAD

- 9 ounces (255 g) spinach leaves, chopped

- 3 eggs, hardboiled, peeled, and chopped into small pieces

- 1 medium-size tomato, chopped

- 1 to 2 avocados, stones removed and flesh scooped out of shell and sliced

- 10 olives, pitted and finely chopped

- 1/4 to 1/2 cup (30 to 60 g) grated Cheddar cheese

- 1/4 cup (60 g) cooked and finely chopped SCD-safe bacon (see chart on pages 17–18)

ANGIE'S VINAIGRETTE

- 1/3 cup (80 ml) olive oil

- 2 to 4 tablespoons (30 to 60 ml) Mock Balsamic Vinegar (page 175)

- 1 tablespoon (15 ml) red wine vinegar

- 1 tablespoon (15 g) ground mustard

- 1 tablespoon (20 g) honey

- 1 orange, juiced

- Salt and ground pepper to taste

To make the salad, toss together the spinach leaves, eggs, tomato, and avocados in salad bowl. Sprinkle the top of the salad with the olives, cheese, and bacon bits.

To make the vinaigrette, combine all the ingredients thoroughly, until they dissolve into each other, especially the mustard. Toss with the salad and serve.

YIELD: Salad makes 5 to 7 servings; vinaigrette makes 1 1/2 cups (350 ml)

Aunt Maggie's Spinach Salad and Uncle Rick's Dressing

Both my Aunt Maggie and my Uncle Rick have artistic personalities—they were always drawing, pasting, cutting, or building projects together during my visits to their home when I was a child. This recipe is a result of their creative collaboration in the kitchen.

INGREDIENTS

SALAD

- 9 ounces (255 g) spinach leaves
- 1 endive
- 1 cup (100 g) grated Manchego cheese

DRESSING

- 2 tablespoons (30 ml) white wine vinegar
- 3 tablespoons (60 g) honey
- 1 tablespoon (15 ml) extra virgin olive oil
- 1/4 cup (40 g) peeled and chopped shallots
- 1/8 teaspoon salt
- 1/8 teaspoon pepper

To make the salad, chop the spinach and endive leaves to the desired size. Sprinkle the cheese on top.

To make the dressing, blend all the dressing ingredients together in a food processor until smooth. Toss with the salad and serve.

YIELD: Salad makes 4 to 6 servings; salad dressing makes 1/3 cup (80 ml)

Fresh Salad with Chunky Olive-Tomato Dressing

The prevalence of tomatoes and olives in both the salad and the dressing provide a strong, consistent flavor.

INGREDIENTS

SALAD

- 9 ounces (255 g) mesclun mix
- 1 1/4 cups (70 g) SCD-safe sun-dried tomatoes (see chart on pages 17–18)
- 3 kalamata olives, pitted and finely chopped
- 1 large cucumber, peeled and sliced into rounds
- 3 large carrots, peeled and sliced into rounds
- 1 red bell pepper, seeded and chopped

DRESSING

- 4 cloves garlic, mashed
- 18 kalamata olives, pitted and chopped
- 1/2 cup (120 ml) olive oil
- 1 1/2 large tomatoes, finely chopped
- 5 tablespoons (80 ml) red wine vinegar
- Salt and pepper to taste

To make the salad, toss together all the ingredients in a salad bowl.

To make the dressing, combine all the ingredients in a small bowl. Toss with the salad, and serve.

YIELD: Salad makes 6 to 7 servings; dressing makes 2 1/2 to 3 cups (590 to 705 ml)

NOTE: The dressing will keep in the refrigerator for about 2 weeks.

Greek Salad

The Greek salad has become such an everyday item in the regular American repertoire, that we almost forget what makes it so special—fresh, crunchy tomatoes and good-quality gourmet olives. An organic or good-quality olive oil and vinegar also make a difference.

INGREDIENTS

- 1 orange bell pepper, finely chopped
- 1/2 large cucumber, peeled and finely chopped
- 1/2 red onion, peeled and finely chopped
- 20 SCD-safe black olives, finely chopped fine (see chart on pages 17–18)
- 2 Roma tomatoes, finely chopped
- 1/4 cup (30 g) crumbled blue cheese, or to taste

DRESSING

- 1 1/2 teaspoons red wine vinegar
- 3/4 teaspoon olive oil

Combine all the ingredients in a salad bowl, except the vinegar and olive oil.

When you are ready to serve, add in those remaining ingredients, and toss the salad.

YIELD: 4 servings

NOTE: The blue cheese has a very strong aftertaste—you can replace it with dry curd cottage cheese, if desired. (Feta cheese, traditionally used in Greek salads, contains too much lactose and is therefore not allowed on the diet.)

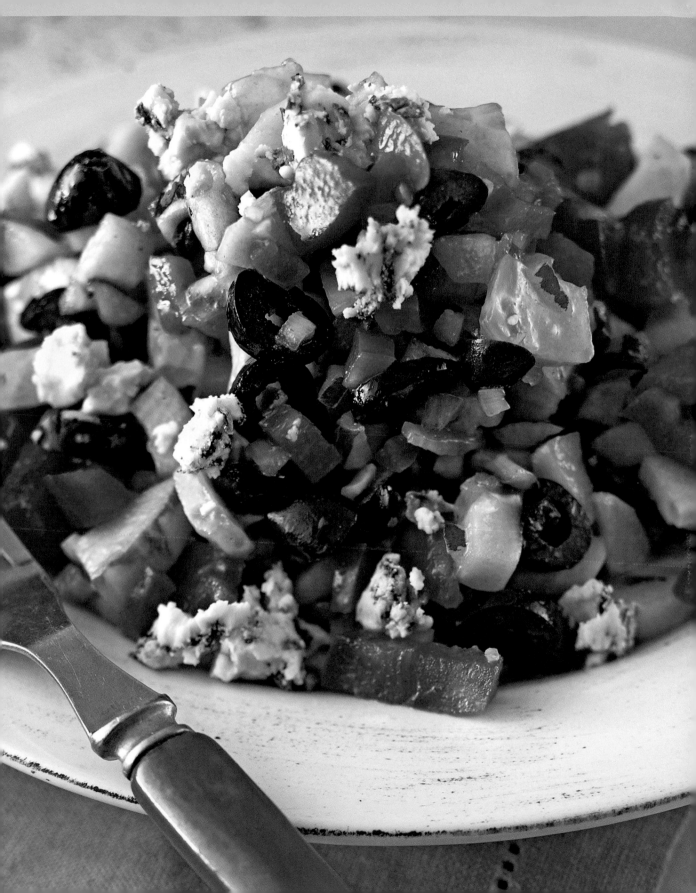

Israeli Carrot Salad

This salad is quick and easy to make, and has a sweet citrus flavor from the oranges.

INGREDIENTS

- 4 large carrots, peeled and grated
- 1/3 cup (50 g) organic seedless raisins
- 3/4 cup (175 ml) freshly squeezed orange juice (use juice oranges, if possible)

Place the grated carrots in a bowl. Add the raisins and orange juice. Mix thoroughly and serve.

YIELD: 4 to 6 servings

NOTE: The orange juice keeps the carrots moistened with flavor. If your carrots are too dry, add more juice as necessary.

Raman's Surprise Salad

Sometimes mistakes can create beautiful consequences. This recipe was a result of starting with one idea but ending up with another.

INGREDIENTS

- 2 tablespoons (30 ml) red wine vinegar
- 1 tablespoon (15 ml) olive oil
- 1 tablespoon (20 g) honey
- 1/2 teaspoon salt
- 1 rib celery, finely diced
- 1 scallion, thinly sliced
- 1 carrot, grated
- 1 Gala apple, cored, peeled, and diced

Whisk together the red wine vinegar, olive oil, honey, and salt in a small bowl. Mix in the celery, scallion, carrot, and apple. Serve immediately or cover and refrigerate.

YIELD: 4 to 6 servings

Spanish Orange-Radish Salad

We initially tried this recipe without the salad leaves, but found the flavor was too concentrated. By introducing the leaves, we softened the impact of the strong citrus punch, the crunchiness of the radishes, and the spiciness of the cumin. It is great as a cooling summer creation—after a day at the beach or a long bike ride on a wooded trail.

INGREDIENTS

- 2 tablespoons (30 ml) extra virgin olive oil
- 3 tablespoons (45 ml) freshly squeezed orange juice
- ¼ teaspoon ground cumin powder
- One 9-ounce (255 g) package or container mesclun salad greens
- 4 oranges, peeled, skinned, and sliced into pieces
- 4 radishes, thinly sliced
- 12 black olives, pitted and cut into strips

Whisk together the olive oil, orange juice, and cumin in a bowl. Set aside.

When you are ready to serve, combine the mesclun salad greens, orange pieces, radishes, and olives in a large salad bowl. Drizzle the dressing over the top, and toss the salad. Serve immediately.

YIELD: 6 to 8 servings

Wilted Mesclun with Portobello Mushrooms

We inherited this recipe from a member of my family during our Christmas visit. The idea of wilting greens sounded a bit odd at first, but once the dish came out of the oven, we could not stop devouring it—it was gone within a matter of minutes.

INGREDIENTS

- 2 ½ tablespoons (38 ml) olive oil, divided
- 4 portobello mushroom caps
- ⅛ teaspoon salt
- Black pepper to taste
- 2 cloves garlic

- 2 vine-ripened tomatoes
- 2 tablespoons Mock Balsamic Vinegar (page 175)
- 3 ½ ounces (100 g) mesclun salad greens
- 3 ounces (85 g) dry curd cottage cheese

Preheat the oven to broil. Use 1 tablespoon (15 ml) of the olive oil to grease an ovenproof baking dish. Place the portobello mushroom caps in the dish, face up, and coat with the oil from the dish, then sprinkle with salt and pepper. Place in the oven and broil for approximately 5 minutes.

Meanwhile, chop the garlic and tomatoes. Remove the mushrooms from the oven, and add the tomatoes and garlic on top of each cap. Drizzle the caps with 1 tablespoon of the remaining olive oil (15 ml) and the balsamic vinegar, distributing evenly among the mushrooms. Place the mushrooms back in the oven, and broil until the mushrooms are tender, approximately 10 minutes. Remove and set aside.

Lightly rub a large ovenproof platter with the remaining ½ tablespoon (8 ml) of olive oil. Scatter the greens on the platter (do not heap them) and place the portobello caps on top of the greens. Sprinkle the dry curd cottage cheese across the platter. Place in the oven for 30 seconds to 1 minute to wilt the greens. Serve immediately.

YIELD: 4 servings

NOTE: Be careful not to leave the greens in the oven too long or they will turn brown and lose their flavor.

CHAPTER 5

Snacks

After a trip to Rajasthan, India—walking through ancient castles, examining intricate miniature paintings, seeing seventeenth-century swords designed for one-handed use that most people could move only with both hands, and viewing the clothes of an ancient king reputed to be 7 feet tall and 400 pounds—I came away thinking that perhaps if J. R. R. Tolkien had visited this place, he wouldn't have had to stretch his imagination quite so much.

During my trip I had snacks in my backpack and even stored yogurt back in the hotel refrigerator. But one of the modern kings of Rajasthan traveled heavier than I ever did; For his 1902 tour of Britain, Maharaja Madhao Singh II refused to use water from any other (especially English) sources: only the holy Ganges River water would suit his needs. So for his trip, he commissioned two giant silver containers to be built so that he could carry the Ganges water abroad. Each stood 5-foot 3-inches, weighed 681 pounds, and held more than 237 gallons of water.

I pointed this out to my wife, Nilou: "See, I'm not the only one carrying around my own supplies!"

Avocado on Tomato

This is a very simple, quick snack. It does not require more than a few minutes to make, but will provide maximum satisfaction. You can enjoy it in any season and any location, as long as you have 5 minutes to spare.

INGREDIENTS

- 1 large tomato
- 1 avocado
- 1 teaspoon lime juice
- Salt and pepper to taste

Cut the tomato into thick, round slices and place on a plate. Scoop out the avocado in a separate small bowl, and mash until soft. Add the lime juice, salt, and pepper to the bowl, and mix well.

Place a portion of the mixture on top of the tomato slices. Enjoy!

YIELD: 5 to 7 slices

Banana-Poppy Treat

This quick snack will make you feel very happy that you are on the SCD!

INGREDIENTS

- 1 tablespoon (14 g) butter
- 2 teaspoons poppy seeds*
- 1 tablespoon (20 g) honey
- 1 large ripe banana, sliced into rounds

Melt the butter in a small stovetop pan, add the poppy seeds, and sauté for 1 to 2 minutes. Add the honey, and stir until it is absorbed into the butter, approximately 1 minute.

Finally, add in the banana slices, and cover them in the poppy-honey-butter sauce. Cook for 2 to 3 minutes, until they soften (but don't let them become mushy). Enjoy plain, or with a dollop of SCD Yogurt (page 19).

YIELD: 1 serving

*NOTE: Wait at least three months after symptoms have cleared before trying seeds.

Citrus-Lime Popsicle Sticks

You can replace the orange juice in this recipe with other fruit juices you prefer, such as watermelon or apple. Enjoy it on a hot summer's day!

INGREDIENTS

- 1 ½ cups (350 ml) freshly squeezed orange juice
- 1 lime, juiced
- 1 teaspoon honey

Stir all the ingredients together, until the honey has melted into the juices.

Remove any citrus seeds; pulp can remain, as it will add to the texture of the popsicle.

Pour into popsicle molds.

Freeze for 3 to 4 hours, or until frozen.

YIELD: 4 popsicles

Mumbai Street Snack

This ubiquitous Indian snack, called bhel in Mumbai, can be bought from the street-corner vendor—a tasty spicy delight for a few rupees. Here is an SCD version of it, which can be tossed together in a few minutes.

INGREDIENTS

- ½ cup (55 g) almond slivers
- 1 tablespoon (10 g) finely chopped red onion
- ½ teaspoon salt
- Pinch of chili powder
- 1 teaspoon fresh cilantro, chopped
- 1 tablespoon (15 ml) fresh lime juice

Mix all the ingredients together in a bowl. Enjoy!

YIELD: 1 serving

NOTE: Eat this snack immediately; otherwise, the lime juice will dampen the almond slivers.

Mixed Nut Brittle

You can make this brittle as a great alternative to store-bought granola and fruit bars. This one is wholesome and filled with real ingredients.

INGREDIENTS

- 1 cup (150 g) cashews
- 2 cups (300 g) shelled pistachios
- 1 cup (100 g) walnuts
- 2 cups (215 g) almond slivers
- 1 1/2 cups (510 g) honey
- 1 1/2 sticks (190 g) butter

Preheat the oven to 325°F (170°C, or gas mark 3).

Dry-roast or toast all the nuts by spreading them on a baking tray and baking until dark golden brown, 15 to 20 minutes. Allow the nuts to cool and then mix them well in a bowl.

In a large saucepan, heat the honey until it simmers, then add the butter. Whisk it into the honey until the mixture becomes sauce-like in consistency. These two steps will take about 5 minutes. Remove the sauce-pan from the heat and stir in the nuts until they are thoroughly coated with the mixture. Pour the mixture into a 9- by 13-inch (23- by 33-cm) baking pan, spreading it out evenly.

Place the pan in the freezer for 1 to 1 1/2 hours. Make sure the brittle becomes hard and can be cut with a knife. Remove from the freezer, cut the brittle into small squares, wrap each one individually in waxed paper, and return to the freezer for storage.

YIELD: Twenty to twenty-five 2-inch squares

NOTE: You can use other nuts in this recipe if you prefer.

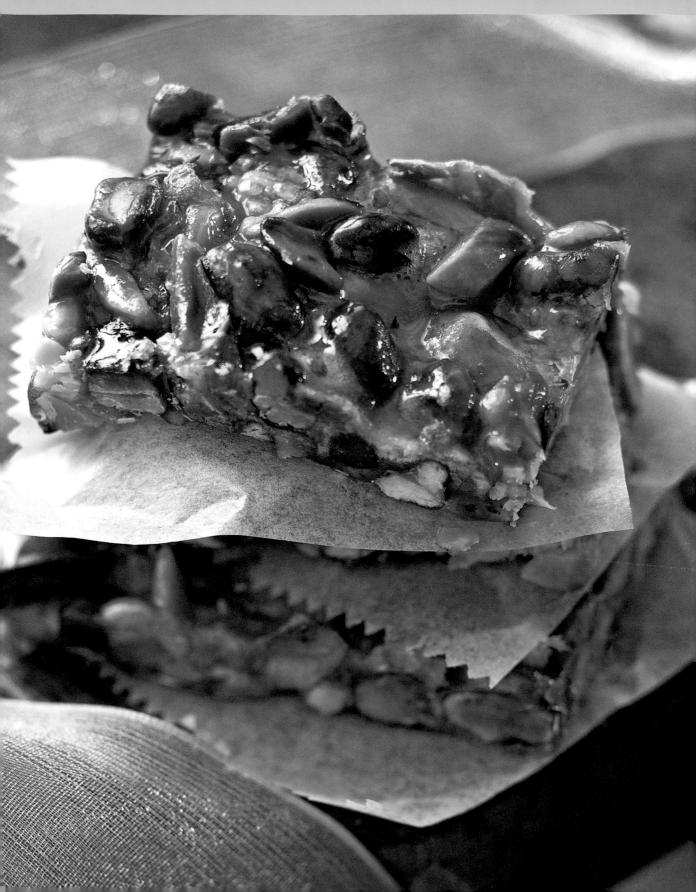

Nut Cheese Balls

This quick snack may be enjoyed on top of tomato slices.

INGREDIENTS

- ½ cup (115 g) dry curd cottage cheese
- ⅛ teaspoon salt
- ⅛ teaspoon oregano
- ⅛ teaspoon thyme
- ¼ cup (35 g) pine nuts
- 1 teaspoon Spiced Butter/Ghee (page 178) or butter

In a bowl, combine the cheese, spices, and nuts. (The mixture will resemble a giant ball.) Form into 15 small balls, approximately ¼ inch (6 mm) in size.

In a medium-size, nonstick skillet, melt the Spiced Butter/Ghee over medium heat and place the balls in the pan for 30 seconds to 1 minute, rolling them around to make sure they absorb the butter.

Using a spatula, remove the nut cheese balls from the pan, transfer to a plate, and let cool.

YIELD: 15 nut cheese balls

NOTE: The heat causes the cheese to become slightly moist and stringy, which holds the mixture together.

Radha's Masala Nut Mix

My father came to the United States from India in his early twenties and achieved the immigrant's dream—a house in the suburbs, a good job, eventual retirement, and the benefits that come with it. One of these benefits is time to relax. On some evenings, he takes to watching new and old Hindi movies, and reminiscing about his childhood in India. These Bollywood films, along with his favorite masala nuts below, allow him to revisit long-forgotten memories of friends and family there.

INGREDIENTS

- 1 cup (100 g) chopped pecans
- 1/2 cup (50 g) chopped walnuts
- 1/2 cup (46 g) sliced almonds
- 1 cup (150 g) cashews
- 1/2 teaspoon peanut oil
- 1 teaspoon salt
- 1/2 teaspoon chili powder
- 1/2 teaspoon white pepper

Mix all the ingredients together. Store in an airtight container.

YIELD: 3 1/2 cups (400 g)

NOTE: Do not purchase nuts in salted mixtures because they often include starch.

Raman's Trail Mix

Trail mix is a great snack, especially when traveling. You can use the nuts in different proportions, depending on which specific ones you prefer.

INGREDIENTS

- 2 cups (200 g) walnuts
- 2 cups (200 g) pecans
- 1 cup (150 g) Brazil nuts
- 1 cup (150 g) hazelnuts
- 1 cup (92 g) sliced almonds
- 1 cup (150 g) shelled pistachios
- 2 cups (290 g) raisins
- 1 cup (175 g) SCD-safe dates, chopped into bits (see chart on pages 17–18)
- 1 cup (175 g) SCD-safe dried apricots, chopped into bits (see chart on pages 17–18)

Coarsely chop the walnuts, pecans, Brazil nuts, and hazelnuts together (you can use a dull blade on a food processor to do this), so that they are not totally pulverized, but still chunky. Remove from the processor, add all the remaining ingredients, and combine. Store the mixture in an airtight container.

YIELD: 12 cups (1600 g)

Tricolor Chips

Snacking on a bag of potato chips is a long-forgotten dream for a lot of us on the SCD, but this recipe more than makes up for that longing!

INGREDIENTS

- 2 carrots
- 1 beet
- 1 celeriac root
- Olive oil for deep-frying
- Salt to taste (optional)

Peel the carrots, beet, and celeric root and cut them into paper-thin slices.

In a large wok or deep frying pan, pour in the oil ½ to 1 inch deep (1.3 to 2.5 cm), and allow it to heat until crackling. Add the chips to the heated oil, and fry them until crisp, 5 to 10 minutes. Usually only a single layer of chips will fit for frying in the pan, so you might need to do a couple of batches (you can reuse the same oil). Layer a plate with absorbent napkins, and when the chips are done, place them on the plate so the paper absorbs the excess oil.

Toss with salt, if desired, and serve immediately.

YIELD: 1 to 2 servings

CHAPTER 6

Appetizers

My friend Frank and I sat in a small, white, insect-encrusted car on the outskirts of Sevilla, Spain. In front of us stood a closed gate. On the opposite side stood five bulls, the nearest 20 yards away. All of them stared at us. The dirt road beyond them led to our destination, a bank on the Guadiamar River. Careful not to drop our gazes from the bulls, we discussed options.

Me: "I know your university needs that water sample, but at some of our prior locations the river bed was dry. We can just say that there was no water here."

Frank: "These measurements are important for the river's restoration. They have to be taken at the same location each year. We have to go to that bank."

Me: "Yeah, but the bulls are between us and the river."

Frank: "This is about scientific integrity... nevermind. Just think of the food we'll have after this is over instead."

Me: "I'll get the gate."

Kicking up dust, I unlocked the gate, swung it open, and dove back to the car. When the car started forward, the bulls briefly stood their ground. But we were soon able to breath again when they scattered out of sight. Shortly after collecting the samples, we headed back to the city. There we'd made a habit of happily ordering plates of tapas and watching the Euro Cup on the TVs at the local restaurants.

This section contains some favorite tapas recipes (appetizers) from different parts of the globe.

Grilled Asparagus with Tangy Dip

This tapas recipe has its roots in Spanish cuisine. It is a blend of a simple green that is grilled or broiled to bring out its delicate flavor, and then complemented with a strong, flavor-infused nutty vinaigrette.

INGREDIENTS

ASPARAGUS

- 1 pound (455 g) asparagus
- 1 tablespoon (15 ml) olive oil

DIP

- 1 ½ tablespoons (21 g) butter
- 1 cup (100 g) walnuts
- 2 tablespoons (30 ml) olive oil
- ¼ cup (60 ml) red wine vinegar
- 3 tablespoons (60 g) honey
- 1 teaspoon mustard powder
- ¼ teaspoon salt
- ¼ cup (60 ml) water, or more as needed

To make the asparagus, preheat the oven to broil. Cut the bottom ends off the asparagus. Coat a baking dish with 1 tablespoon (15 ml) of the olive oil, and place the asparagus in it. Rub the oil onto the asparagus. Broil until cooked, 10 to 15 minutes. Transfer to a serving plate.

To make the dip, melt 1 tablespoon of the butter in a skillet over low heat. Add the walnuts and sauté until the walnuts are slightly browned, approximately 2 minutes. Be careful not to allow them to burn. Set aside.

Meanwhile, in a food processor, combine all the remaining ingredients (including the remaining butter) for the dip, then add the toasted walnuts. Blend until it is a smooth purée. If you would like a thinner dip, add additional tablespoons of water until you've reached the desired consistency.

Spoon the dip over the asparagus on the plate, or set aside in a dipping bowl (depending on the consistency).

YIELD: 3 to 4 servings

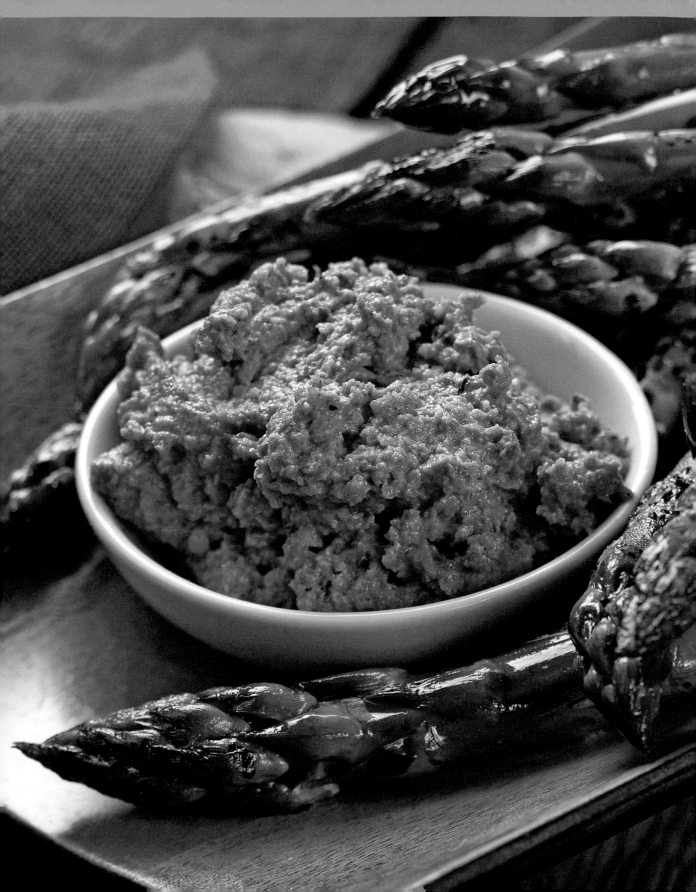

Chicken Satay

Indonesia, an archipelago of more than 15,000 islands, is often heralded as the originator of satay—a marinade that can be applied to many meats. Nowadays, you can find this signature appetizer in almost any part of the world, but this SCD-friendly version is only specific to our cookbook.

INGREDIENTS

SATAY MARINADE

- 1 teaspoon whole coriander seeds*
- 1 teaspoon whole cumin seeds*
- 4 cloves garlic, finely minced
- 3/4 to 1 tablespoon (5 to 6 g) peeled and grated fresh ginger
- 1 tablespoon (8 g) Curry Powder (page 175)
- 1/16 teaspoon turmeric powder
- 1/2 cup (120 ml) SCD Coconut Milk* (page 177)
- 2 tablespoons (40 g) honey

- 1 pound (455 g) flattened chicken cutlets, cut into 1-inch (2.5-cm) cubes
- 1 teaspoon olive oil

To make the marinade, toast (dry-roast) the coriander and cumin seeds in small pan for 1 to 2 minutes, and then pulverize them in a spice grinder, or crush them using a mortar and pestle. In a large bowl, whisk together all the marinade ingredients, including the seed mixture, until well mixed.

Add the chicken cubes to the marinade, and allow to marinate for 1 hour.

When you are ready to cook the satay, heat the olive oil in a skillet on the stovetop, and cook the chicken until done. Baste the chicken with the marinade so it does not dry out. You could also cook this dish on an outdoor grill.

YIELD: 3 to 4 servings

NOTE: You can buy flattened chicken cutlets at the grocery store, but you can also flatten regular chicken breasts at home.

*NOTE: Wait at least three months after symptoms have cleared before trying seeds. Wait at least six months after symptoms have cleared before trying coconut milk.

Kiwi Appetizer

This simple Chilean appetizer takes 5 to 10 minutes to prepare for a quick hors d'oeuvre served with cocktails. The saltiness and sweetness weave together in a way that is surprising, but pleasant.

INGREDIENTS

- 3 kiwifruit
- ½ large cucumber
- 8 thin slices SCD-safe prosciutto (see chart on pages 17–18)
- 8 toothpicks
- 1 lime, juiced

Peel the kiwifruit, and cut into round slices approximately ¼ inch (6 mm) thick, which should yield 16 slices total. Set aside. Peel the cucumber, and cut into round slices the same thickness as the kiwi. The cucumber should yield 8 slices.

Make a "sandwich" with the kiwi and cucumber slices by placing 1 cucumber slice in between 2 kiwi slices. Then take 1 thin slice of prosciutto and wrap it around the "sandwich." Secure it with a toothpick so it holds together. Repeat this for all the remaining kiwi and cucumber slices and prosciutto. This process should yield 8 wrapped "sandwiches."

Brush the sandwiches with the lime juice, and serve.

YIELD: 4 servings

NOTE: As an alternative, you can withhold the cucumbers and use only the kiwi and prosciutto.

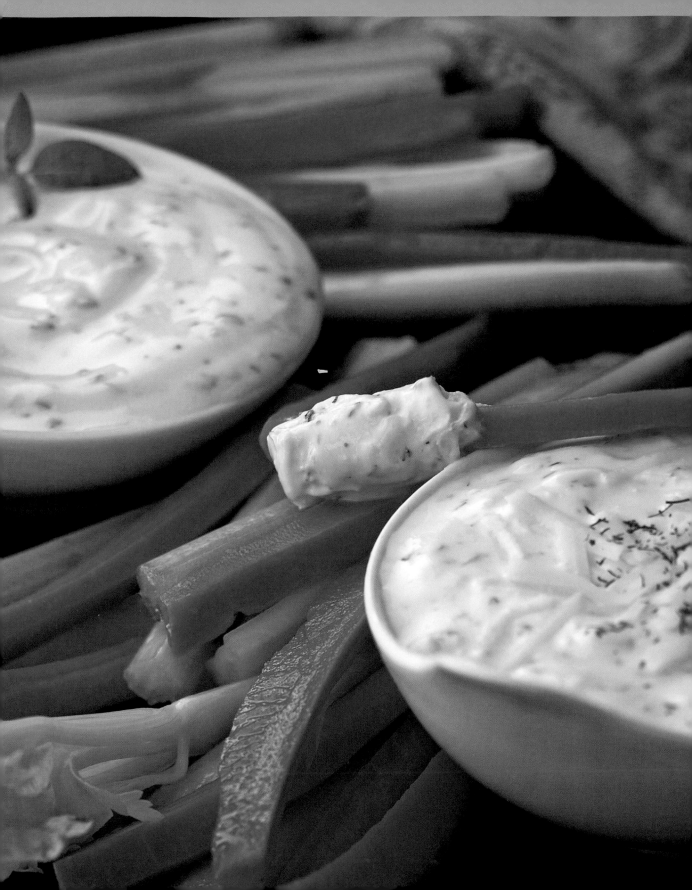

Herb Dips with Veggie Sticks

The yogurt cheese creates a creamy consistency that can be used for all sorts of dip variations. Below are two variations that we thought were flavorful—you can modify these and add your own selection of herb preferences to this recipe.

INGREDIENTS

VEGGIE STICKS

- 2 to 3 large carrots
- 2 to 3 large celery stalks

DILL DIP

- 6 tablespoons (85 g) Yogurt Cheese (page 182)
- 1 teaspoon Parmesan cheese, grated
- 1/2 teaspoon dried dill
- 1/2 teaspoon salt
- 2 cloves garlic, peeled and mashed

OREGANO AND THYME DIP

- 6 tablespoons (85 g) Yogurt Cheese (page 182)
- 1/2 teaspoon salt
- 1/4 teaspoon black pepper
- 1/4 teaspoon oregano
- 1/4 teaspoon thyme

To make the veggie sticks, peel the carrots. Cut both the carrots and the celery vertically into long narrow sticks for easy dipping.

To make the dips, mix the ingredients for each dip separately with the yogurt, so that you create two distinct dips. Add more yogurt cheese to the mixture(s) if you feel the flavors are too strong.

Place the dips in two bowls in the center of a plate, and arrange the celery and carrots around.

YIELD: 8 to 10 servings

Gourmet Burgerettes

This mini version of the traditional American burger will allow you to eat more than one with abandon! The Tricolor Chips (page 76) and Minty Limeade (page 208) complement this dish for a nice Fourth of July celebration.

INGREDIENTS

- 2 eggs
- 3/4 teaspoon cracked black pepper
- 3/4 teaspoon dried basil
- 1/2 cup (55 g) almond flour
- 2 ounces (55 g) Cheddar cheese, grated
- 1 pound (455 g) ground beef
- Olive oil

Preheat the oven to 350°F (180°C, or gas mark 4). Lightly grease a large ovenproof tray with olive oil.

In a small bowl, combine the eggs, black pepper, basil, almond flour, and cheese. Add the mixture to the ground beef, and knead until everything is fully combined.

Make small, 1/2-inch (1.3-cm) balls of the meat mixture. Place them on the greased tray and flatten them into thin mini-meat patties.

Lightly brush the tops of the patties with olive oil (so the patties don't dry out in the oven).

Cook in the oven until the underside is cooked through, 10 to 15 minutes. Flip and cook the other side.

Remove from the oven and allow to cool.

YIELD: 20 to 30 mini burgers, depending on size

Ludovico Cabbage Dumplings

We got this recipe from old friends of the family, Tom and Mary, who have spent the last few Thanksgivings with us. This recipe has roots in Eastern Europe, but has been modified for the SCD.

INGREDIENTS

- 1 teaspoon olive oil
- 1 large onion, finely chopped
- 3 cloves garlic, peeled and finely chopped
- 1 pound (455 g) ground beef
- Salt and pepper to taste
- 6 dates, pitted and finely chopped
- 1 medium-size cabbage

Heat the olive oil in a stovetop pan and add the onion and garlic. When they are browned (4 to 5 minutes), add the beef, salt, and pepper. Sauté the beef until it is cooked halfway through. Add the chopped dates, and let the beef cook until done, 15 to 20 minutes. Remove from the heat and set aside.

Meanwhile, bring a pot of water to a boil. Separate the cabbage leaves (peel the cabbage to keep each full leaf intact). Drop each leaf into the water, and boil until they become pliable (the leaves will turn slightly transparent), 3 to 5 minutes. Remove them from the water, and set aside.

Preheat the oven to 350°F (180°C, or gas mark 4).

Heap a bit of the beef mixture into the center of each cabbage leaf, and wrap it up. Secure it with a toothpick, if necessary. Place the "rolled" cabbage leaves in a baking dish, and bake in the oven for 5 to 10 minutes. (This is mainly to get rid of excess water in the cabbage leaves from the boiling.)

Serve immediately.

YIELD: 12 to 15 rolls, depending on size of roll

Shrimp Seviche

Seviche, also known as cebiche or ceviche, has its roots in South America. In the last few decades it has gained universal appeal across South and Central America, extending to Costa Rica, Panama, Ecuador, and Mexico. We have chosen to use shrimp for our particular recipe, although in other versions you can use other seafood, such as octopus or white fish.

INGREDIENTS

- 1 pound (455 g) shrimp, peeled and deveined
- 2 tablespoons (36 g) salt
- 3 limes, juiced
- 3 lemons, juiced
- 1 serrano chile
- 1/2 small red onion, peeled
- 1/2 cucumber, peeled
- 1/2 stick celery
- 1 Roma tomato
- 1/4 cup (15 g) fresh cilantro, chopped

Bring 1 to 2 quarts (1.1 to 2.2 litres) of water to boil in a deep pot on the stovetop, and add the shrimp and salt. Allow the shrimp to cook for 3 to 5 minutes, or until done. Do not allow it to overcook, as the shrimp will turn rubbery. Remove the shrimp from the water and place in a bowl with ice so they cool down immediately and stop cooking.

Remove the tails from the shrimp, and slice the shrimp horizontally (down the center) into 2 halves. Chop the shrimp into smaller pieces, if desired. Put the cut shrimp in a glass bowl, add the citrus juices, and mix together. Cover the bowl with plastic wrap and place in the refrigerator for 30 minutes.

Meanwhile, remove the spine and seeds from the chile and chop into very fine pieces. Chop the red onion, cucumber, celery, and tomato and set aside. Mix all the chopped items into the bowl that has the shrimp, and chill in the refrigerator for another 30 minutes.

When ready to serve, add the freshly chopped cilantro.

YIELD: 4 to 6 servings

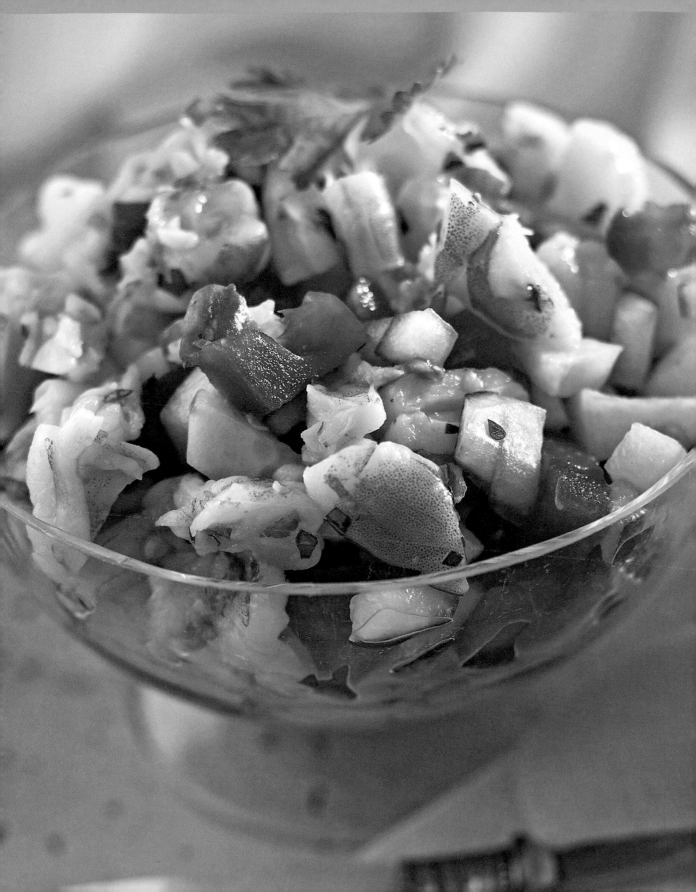

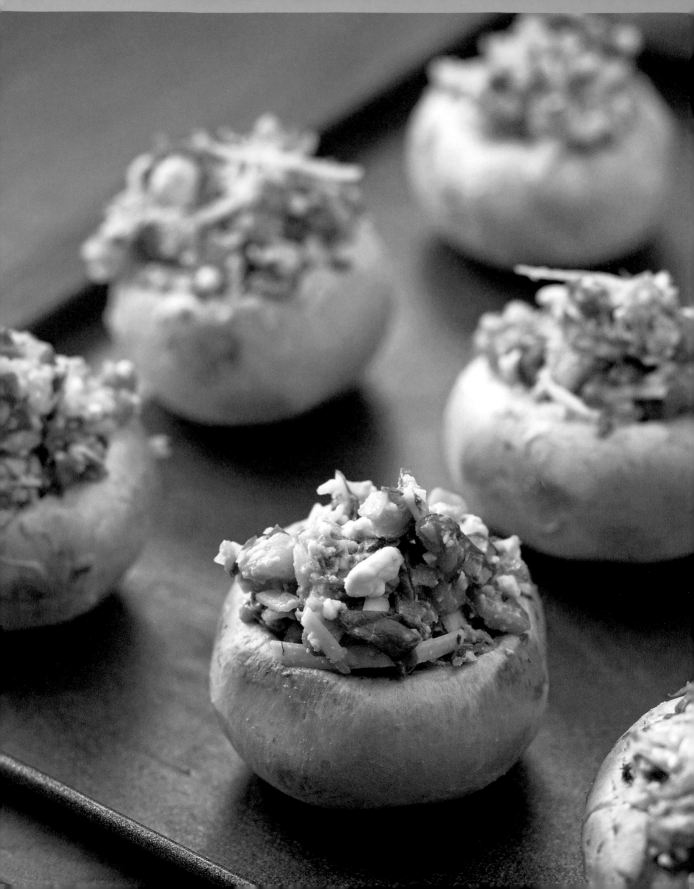

Sue's Stuffed Mushrooms

My mom often makes this recipe as an appetizer when the family gets together. The mushrooms are quite addictive, as it is easy to keep popping them into your mouth.

INGREDIENTS

- 1 pound (455 g) white mushrooms
- 4 ounces (115 g) fresh chopped spinach
- 3 ounces (85 g) dry curd cottage cheese
- 4 cloves garlic, finely minced
- 1 egg
- 1/8 to 1/4 cup (13 to 26 g) grated Parmesan cheese
- 1/4 teaspoon salt

Preheat the oven to 400°F (200°C, or gas mark 6).

Clean the mushrooms. Separate the mushroom stems and caps. Set the caps aside.

Chop up the stems. In a bowl, combine the mushroom stems with the remaining ingredients.

Place the mushroom caps on an ovenproof tray. Heap the mixture from the bowl into each cap. Bake on the top shelf of the oven for 15 minutes.

YIELD: 4 to 6 servings

Haidy's Zucchini Canoes

We were given this recipe by a Venezuelan friend of ours, who called the zucchini halves "canoes"!

INGREDIENTS

- 6 green zucchini, 6 to 8 inches (15 to 20 cm) long
- 2 tablespoons (30 ml) olive oil, divided
- 10 cloves garlic, minced
- 1 medium-size onion, finely chopped
- 2 medium-size tomatoes, diced
- 1 1/2 cups (175 g) grated Swiss or Cheddar cheese

Preheat the oven to 350°F (180°C, or gas mark 4).

Cut the zucchini vertically into halves, so that you get two long sides for each. Using a spoon, scoop the inner pulp out of each half and place it in a separate bowl. The result should be boat-like zucchini shells (canoes).

Coat the bottom of a baking dish with 1/2 tablespoon (8 ml) of the olive oil. (Use a baking dish large enough to fit all the halves.) Put the zucchini in the baking dish and use another 1/2 tablespoon (8 ml) of the olive oil to lightly brush the canoes. Place the baking dish in the oven and bake for 15 to 20 minutes.

On the stovetop, in a separate pan, heat the remaining 1 tablespoon (15 ml) of olive oil and sauté the garlic and onion until slightly brown. Next, add in the reserved zucchini pulp and the tomatoes. Sauté them together until soft.

Remove the canoes from the oven, and divide the sautéed stovetop mixture among the canoes. Put the canoes back into the oven for another 15 to 20 minutes, or until the shells begin to soften (it depends on how crunchy you like your zucchini—you can leave it in longer if you like it softer).

Add the grated cheese to the top of each canoe, and place them back into the oven for another 10 to 15 minutes, or until the cheese has melted.

YIELD: 12 zucchini canoes

CHAPTER 7

Side Dishes

Until the age of seventeen, my father grew up in a remote village located in northern India. Like any child, he went to school during the week, and what he looked forward to the most were specially prepared, homecooked meals when he got home.

Everyday staples included rice,* lentils (dal), and yogurt. However, for each meal, two or three additional side dishes would also be served. Made from fresh vegetables grown in a small family garden or in the green fields nearby, these dishes changed with the seasons: squashes and spinach in the winter, radishes in the summer, and string beans and eggplant during monsoon season. Spiced and cooked, the side dishes gave a distinctive flavor to these meals.

Having all meals made from food grown within sight now seems rare. My father hasn't been back to his village home for many years, and when I asked him about those dishes and meals, his eyes lit up in remembrance. But then he thought of another childhood experience that is almost universal: "I also had my least favorite dishes, you know, the ones my mom would make me eat because they were supposed to be good for me."

In creating this section, we hope to take those oft-overlooked and forgotten sides and make them part of our mealtime again!

*NOTE: Rice is not allowed on the diet.

Tasty Brussels Sprouts

This simple, steamed recipe will make you appreciate this often-neglected vegetable—satisfaction guaranteed.

INGREDIENTS

- 20 small or medium-size Brussels sprouts
- 1 tablespoon (14 g) butter
- Salt to taste

To prepare the Brussels sprouts, remove wilted or yellow leaves, wash them, and then remove or cut off the stem base. Halve or quarter each sprout.

Steam the sprouts until they are cooked, approximately 20 to 30 minutes. Melt butter in a stovetop sauté pan and add the sprouts. Cook for several minutes. Add salt, if desired.

YIELD: 2 to 3 servings

Chilean Fruit Salsa

This Chilean dish is usually served as an accompaniment to chicken or fish. We discovered it is also good on its own as an early morning indulgence! The avocado adds in the calories and the fruit packs a healthy punch.

INGREDIENTS

- 2 nectarines
- 1 pear
- 2 apricots
- 1 kiwifruit
- 1 Anaheim chile
- ½ cup (80 g) chopped spring onion
- 1 ripe avocado
- ½ cup (30 g) fresh cilantro, chopped
- ½ lime, juiced

Cut and deseed the nectarines, pear, and apricots and chop into small pieces. Peel the kiwifruit and do the same. Place all the fruit in a bowl. Deseed the chile and chop into very fine pieces. Add the chile and the onion to the fruit bowl. Cut the avocado in half, scoop out the flesh, and add to the mixture. Mix in the chopped cilantro and juice. Toss all the ingredients together until they are thoroughly mixed. Serve immediately.

YIELD: 4 to 6 servings

NOTE: Prepare this dish right before serving, otherwise the avocado will turn brown.

Cubanelle Peppers

This recipe takes about 5 minutes to prepare. The flavors released from the peppers when they are broiled are sweet and delicious. It is a great side dish for a sit-down dinner, or as part of a lunch sandwich.

INGREDIENTS

- 6 to 8 Cubanelle/Italian peppers, cut into chunks
- 2 tablespoons (15 ml) olive oil
- 1 teaspoon salt

Preheat the oven to broil. On a large baking tray, mix together the olive oil and salt so that the tray is coated. Rub all the excess oil (there will be plenty) onto the peppers until they are evenly covered. Broil in the oven until they are soft and slightly browned, but not charred, 20 to 30 minutes.

YIELD: 2 to 4 servings

Polish Sauerkraut

This sauerkraut does not require any fermentation—it is a fresh stovetop version that should be eaten immediately. It goes well with Simple Pork Roast (page 152).

INGREDIENTS

- ½ medium onion, chopped
- ½ teaspoon caraway seeds*
- ½ tablespoon butter
- ½ medium-size cabbage, grated
- 1 apple, cored, peeled, and chopped
- 1 cup (235 ml) water
- ⅛ cup (30 ml) cider vinegar
- 1 teaspoon honey

In a large pot, sauté the onion and caraway seeds in butter until softened and browned, about 5 to 7 minutes. Remove from the pot and set aside. Add all the other ingredients to the pot. Bring to a boil and then simmer on low for 45 minutes.

Do not allow the ingredients to dry out completely. Alternatively, if there is excess water, boil it down so that the sauerkraut is not floating in it. Stir in the onion mixture and serve.

YIELD: 4 to 5 servings

***NOTE:** Wait at least three months after symptoms have cleared before trying seeds.*

Mango Salsa

The idea of a mango salsa recipe was sent to us by an Indian friend, who is mad about mangoes. We received an almost duplicate version of it from another friend who had tried something similar in the Caribbean area. We are integrating both their ingredients to create a unique SCD version for this book.

INGREDIENTS

- 2 ripe mangoes, peeled and diced
- 1 serrano chile, finely chopped
- 2 spring onions, finely chopped
- 1/2 red pepper, finely chopped
- 1/2 yellow pepper, finely chopped
- 1 cup (60 g) fresh cilantro, finely chopped
- 1 lime, juiced, or more to taste

Place the mango pieces in a bowl. Add in the chopped chile, spring onions, and red and yellow bell peppers.

Mix in the cilantro and lime juice. Add more lime juice if necessary. Allow to sit in the refrigerator for 1 hour before serving.

YIELD: 4 to 6 servings

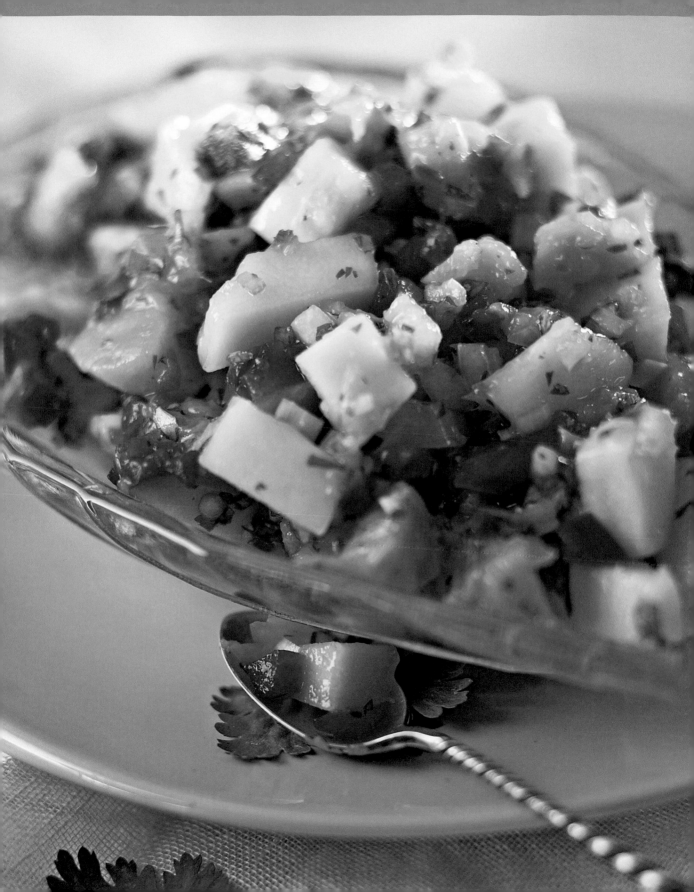

Shilpa's Roasted Beets

The roasting of the beets with the spices releases a warm, rich flavor.

INGREDIENTS

- 2 small to medium-size beets
- 1 tablespoon (15 ml) Mock Balsamic Vinegar (page 175)
- 1 clove garlic, minced
- ¼ teaspoon oregano
- 1 tablespoon (15 ml) olive oil
- Salt and pepper to taste

Preheat the oven to 400°F (200°C, or gas mark 6).

Clean the beets well with the skin on, and then cut into quarters. Combine the remaining ingredients in a small bowl, then toss with the beets. Place the beets on a piece of aluminum foil. Cover and seal the foil (using more foil, if necessary) so that a secure "bag" is created. Bake in the oven until the beets are cooked through, about 1 hour.

YIELD: 1 to 2 servings

Snow Pea Sauté

The crunchiness of the snow peas and bell peppers are a great combination. This is a terrific side for a chicken or fish entrée.

INGREDIENTS

- 2 tablespoons (28 g) butter
- 1 ½ pounds (685 g) snow peas
- 1 red bell pepper, seeded and diced

In a stovetop pan, melt the butter over medium heat.

Add the snow peas and bell pepper, and sauté until the desired doneness is reached. If you prefer the vegetables on the crispy side, you might want to remove the pan earlier; otherwise, let the vegetables cook until softened.

YIELD: 8 to 10 servings

Southeast Asian Bok Choy

My brother, Ravi, became a vegetarian recently. He and his girlfriend were coming over for dinner. I realized that I should be experimenting with more vegetarian SCD recipes, in my goal of providing him with the nutrients he needs on his diet, as well as on mine.

INGREDIENTS

- 2 teaspoons sesame seeds*
- 1 tablespoon (15 ml) sesame oil
- 1 tablespoon (8 g) peeled and freshly grated ginger
- 2 cloves garlic, freshly pressed
- 4 heads baby bok choy
- 2 tablespoons (30 ml) SCD Asian Sauce (page 173)

Dry-roast the sesame seeds in a large frying pan (which you will be using to cook the bok choy). Dry-roasting involves adding the seeds to the pan on medium heat (without any oil) and letting them brown slightly, about 1 to 2 minutes. Once they are golden brown, transfer to a dish and set aside.

Heat the sesame oil in the same frying pan, and sauté the ginger and garlic. Stir-fry for approximately 1 minute, or until browned.

Clean and trim the baby bok choy, and chop into small pieces. Then add them to the pan, and stir-fry for another minute. Lastly, stir in the Asian sauce, and cover and cook for another 2 minutes.

Remove the pan from the stovetop, and mix in the toasted sesame seeds.

YIELD: 3 to 4 servings

NOTE: Be careful not to over-roast the sesame seeds. After roasting, the seeds should be golden brown.

*NOTE: Wait at least three months after symptoms have cleared before trying seeds.

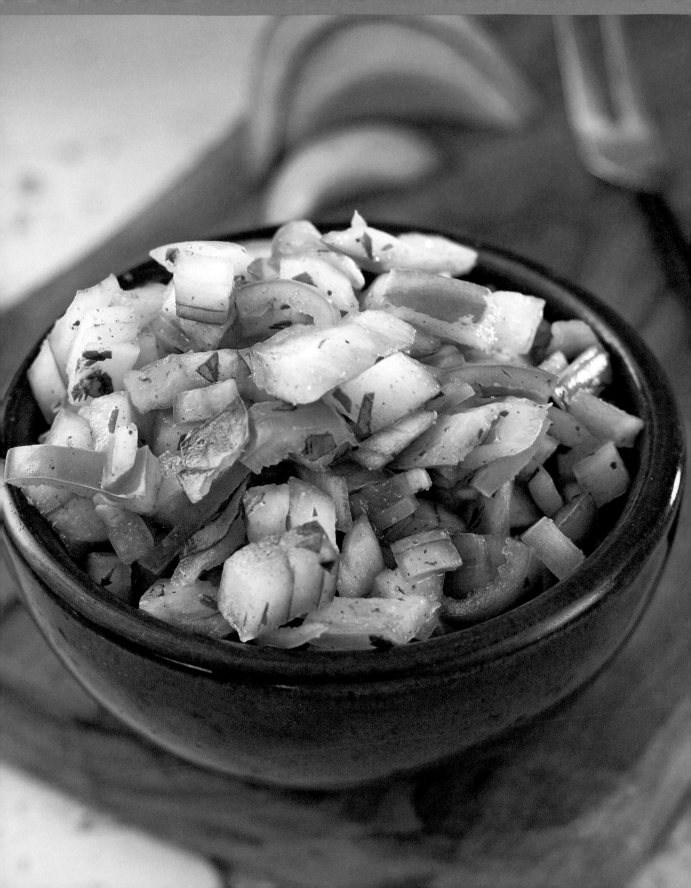

Red Onions with Lime

This basic onion dish is served at many homes across South Asia as a side to traditional meat and vegetarian dishes. It is also a fixture on restaurant tables when one goes out to eat. In our food journeys, we recently discovered that this dish is also popular in Peru, which made us wonder which ingredients traveled from here to there, and back again.

INGREDIENTS

- 3 cups (480 g) finely chopped red onions
- 1 Anaheim chile, seeded and finely chopped
- 2 limes, juiced
- 1 tablespoon (4 g) chopped fresh cilantro, or more to taste
- 1/2 teaspoon salt
- 1/8 teaspoon chili powder
- 1/4 teaspoon cumin powder

Mix together all the ingredients in a bowl, and serve.

YIELD: 6 to 8 servings

Spicy Butternut Squash

Butternut squash is a vine-growing winter squash that has a nutty, warm flavor. The most popular variety of butternut is local to the northeastern United States, and is used often in winter for soups, pies, etc. We have used it often during Thanksgiving as an SCD-friendly alternative to mashed potatoes. In this recipe, we have blended it with roasted garlic and Indian spices to complement its natural sweetness.

INGREDIENTS

- 1 medium-size butternut squash
- 1 tablespoon (14 g) butter, divided
- 2 teaspoons olive oil
- 2 cloves garlic, finely chopped
- 1 dried red chile
- ½ teaspoon mustard seeds*
- ½ teaspoon cumin seeds*
- Salt to taste

Preheat the oven to 400°F (200°C, or gas mark 6).

Peel the squash, cut it in half, and scoop out the inside seeded and stringy area. Place in a baking dish with ½ tablespoon of the butter in the scooped-out areas. Bake until the squash is soft (about 30 to 45 minutes).

In a stovetop pan, heat the olive oil. Add the garlic, red chile, mustard seeds, and cumin seeds. Allow the garlic to brown, and then add the baked squash, mashing it to the consistency you desire. Add the remaining ½ tablespoon butter. Allow to cook for a few minutes until the squash absorbs the spices.

Add salt to taste.

YIELD: 3 to 4 servings

***NOTE:** Wait at least three months after symptoms have cleared before trying seeds.

NOTE: As an alternative, you can steam the squash rather than baking it.

Spinach with Raisins and Nuts

This is a simple-to-cook side dish and one that accompanies fish entrées very well.

INGREDIENTS

- ½ pound (230 g) spinach leaves
- 2 tablespoons (16 g) coarsely chopped walnuts
- ½ tablespoon (7 g) butter
- 4 to 5 spring onions, finely chopped
- 1 teaspoon olive oil
- ½ small red onion, thinly sliced
- 2 cloves garlic, thinly sliced
- ¼ cup (36 g) raisins

Trim and discard the spinach stems, then wash and chop the leaves. Set aside.

In a stovetop pan (that you will eventually use to cook the spinach), roast the walnuts in the butter, about 1 to 2 minutes. Remove them and set aside in a small bowl.

Add the olive oil to the same pan, and when it is heated, sauté the spring onion over low heat for 5 to 10 minutes. Turn up the heat and add the garlic to the pan sauté lightly.

Finally, add the spinach and raisins. Cover and cook for 3 to 5 minutes, or until the spinach wilts. Stir in the reserved walnuts and serve.

YIELD: 2 servings

Squash and Celeriac Home Fries

In this recipe, we tried to replicate the flavors from home fries, but with SCD-safe ingredients. If you want to flavor the home fries differently, add other spices, such as chili powder, oregano, and thyme.

INGREDIENTS

- 1 butternut squash
- 1 large celeriac
- 3 tablespoons (45 ml) olive oil
- 1 to 2 teaspoons salt

Preheat the oven to 350°F (180°C, or gas mark 4).

Peel the butternut squash, cut in half, and scoop out the inside seeds. Chop the squash into $\frac{1}{4}$-inch (6-mm) pieces. Peel the celeriac and chop into small pieces with the excess oil.

Coat a baking tray with olive oil and salt, and coat the celeriac and squash pieces with the excess oil. Make sure all the pieces are coated with the olive oil.

Bake in the oven until browned and cooked through, about 30 to 40 minutes. Turn the fries over during the baking process to ensure that they cook evenly.

YIELD: 2 to 3 servings

NOTE: Celeriac is also known as celery root.

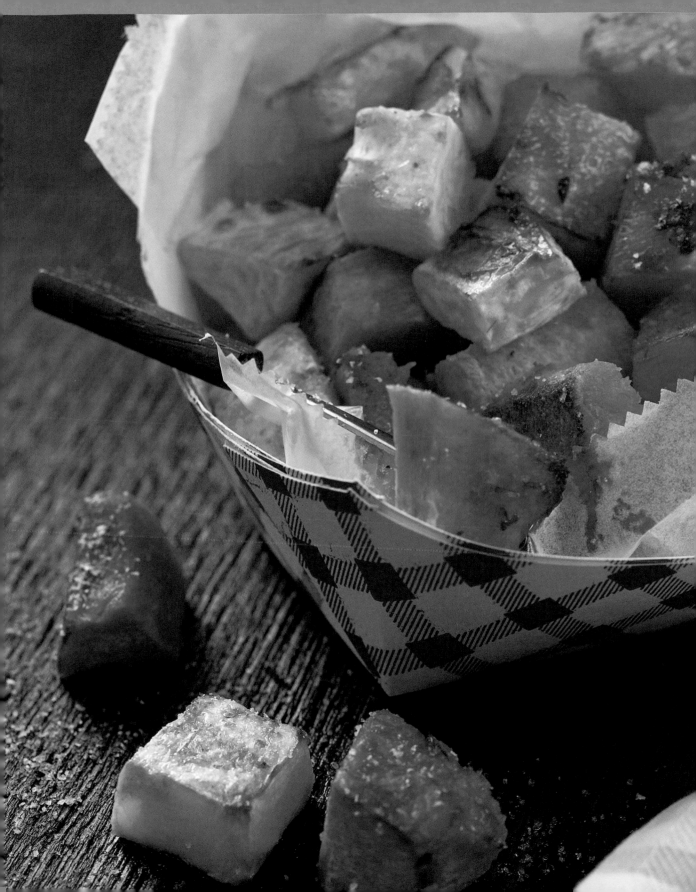

Turkish Baba Ghanoush

My wife and I once had a weekly routine associated with eating baba ghanoush that involved: walking a one-block loop of near our old Brooklyn apartment; ordering takeout with heaps of baba (ghanoush); renting a DVD at the mom-and-pop video rental store; getting a quick drink at the bar while waiting for the takeout; and rushing back home, plopping ourselves in front of the TV, and devouring the food. Over the years, we have moved through many spaces, but the memories of that smoky, creamy baba ghanoush still remain strong.

INGREDIENTS

- 3 large eggplants
- 4 cloves garlic, crushed
- 5 tablespoons (75 g) SCD-safe tahini (see chart on pages 17–18)
- 2 tablespoons (30 ml) olive oil
- 1 lime, juiced
- 1 tablespoon (6 g) fresh mint leaves, finely chopped
- 1 teaspoon salt
- Black pepper to taste

Preheat the oven to 375°F (190°C, or gas mark 5).

Wash the eggplants and pierce them all over with a fork or knife. Transfer to a baking dish.

Roast the eggplants for 45 to 60 minutes, or until they are soft and the skin is blackened. You will need to keep rotating them to make sure they are blackened evenly, and that all sides are cooked through.

Set them aside and allow to cool. Once they come to room temperature, divide each in half and scoop out the inner soft flesh. Discard the blackened skins.

Place the pulp in a food processor with the garlic, tahini, olive oil, lime juice, mint, and salt. Season to taste with pepper. Purée the mixture until it is smooth and creamy.

YIELD: 3 1/2 to 4 cups (790 to 900 g)

CHAPTER 8

Chicken and Other Poultry

My wife and her two sisters have not lived together since the ages of seventeen, twelve, and ten. So now, more than twenty years later, when they are reunited, the preparation and eating of meals becomes an important ritual, one they rarely skip, regardless of one sister having flown halfway around the world the night before, and regardless of jobs, births, deaths, marriages. The sharing of tasks, the talking, and the familiar joking shrink the miles to millimeters, the years and months to mere moments.

Over the years, the dishes cooked have also taken on their own patterns: salads, sides, and soups may come and go, but the one staple of our meals together is a chicken dish. The sisters grew up enjoying their mother's stuffed chicken, and over the years they have had fun creating new variations.

We hope you enjoy some of the recipes they have created in this section.

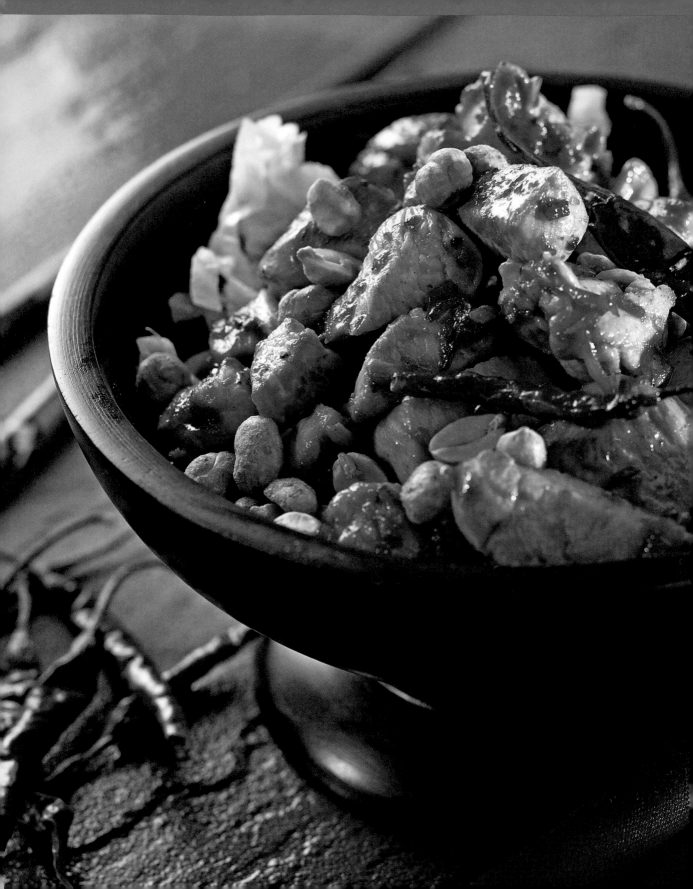

Kung Pao Chicken

Kung Pao chicken is a timeless specialty from central western China. It was first created during the mid-nineteenth century, and gets its name from a governor of the Sichuan Province. In western Chinese restaurants, this dish is symbolic of the culinary skills of the chef. Our SCD version loads up on the peanuts and chiles!

INGREDIENTS

- 5 tablespoons (75 ml) SCD Asian Sauce (page 173)
- 4 cloves garlic, minced
- 2 tablespoons (16 g) grated ginger, divided
- Salt and pepper to taste
- 1 1/4 pounds (570 g) chicken breasts, cubed into 1/2-inch (1.3-cm) pieces
- 1 tablespoon (15 ml) dry white wine
- 1 tablespoon (20 g) honey
- 2 tablespoons (30 ml) sesame oil, divided
- 5 dried chiles
- 1/2 cup (75 g) peanuts

Combine the sauce, garlic, 1 tablespoon (8 g) of the ginger, salt, and pepper in a large bowl. Mix in the chicken pieces and marinate for 30 minutes.

In a separate small bowl, combine the white wine, honey, and 1 tablespoon (15 ml) of the sesame oil. Set aside.

In a wok or stir-fry pan, heat the remaining 1 tablespoon (15 ml) sesame oil. Fry the chiles and remaining 1 tablespoon (8 g) ginger for 1 to 2 minutes, until browned. Next, add the marinated chicken and wine-honey mixture. Cook until the chicken is done, 10 to 15 minutes.

Add the peanuts and toss for 1 minute.

YIELD: 4 to 6 servings

Cape Town Chicken

Cape Town is one of the most beautiful and diverse cities in South Africa. We thought this recipe reflected the unique blend of influences in this region, which come from different parts of Africa, Asia, and Europe.

INGREDIENTS

- 2 limes, juiced
- 1 teaspoon grated lime zest
- ¼ teaspoon salt
- ¼ teaspoon white pepper
- ¼ teaspoon chili powder
- 2 pounds (910 g) boneless chicken breasts, cut into small pieces
- 1 tablespoon (15 ml) olive oil
- 1 red onion, peeled and finely chopped
- 3 cloves garlic, minced
- 2 tomatoes, finely chopped
- 2 teaspoons minced ginger
- 1 cup (235 ml) SCD Coconut Milk* (page 177)

Combine the lime juice and zest, salt, pepper, and chili powder, and marinate the chicken in it for 2 hours.

Heat the olive oil in a stovetop pan. Sauté the red onion and garlic for 5 to 10 minutes on medium heat. Add the marinated chicken and cook until the chicken is almost done, approximately 10 minutes.

Reduce the heat, mix in the tomatoes and ginger, and stir for 3 to 5 minutes.

Finally, pour in the coconut milk and simmer over low heat, stirring frequently, for 10 to 15 minutes, or until the chicken is fully cooked.

YIELD: 6 to 8 servings

*****NOTE:** Wait at least six months after symptoms have cleared before trying coconut milk.

Chicken Curry

A country with more than a dozen official languages, India boasts as much or more variety in its curries. The spices that make up curry differ from region to region. Historically, curry powder is a British creation, an attempt to bottle and define a mixture of different South Asian spices.

INGREDIENTS

- 1 teaspoon olive oil

- 1 onion, chopped

- 4 cloves garlic, minced

- 2 chiles, seeded and chopped

- 1 teaspoon salt

- 1 tablespoon (6 g) minced ginger

- 2 ¹/2 teaspoons Curry Powder (page 175)

- 2 medium-size tomatoes, chopped

- 1 ¹/2 pounds (685 g) chicken breasts, cut into bite-size pieces

- 1 ¹/2 cups (350 ml) water

Heat the olive oil in a pan and sauté the onion, garlic, and chiles for 4 to 5 minutes. Add the salt, ginger, and curry powder and cook for 1 to 2 minutes, stirring to prevent sticking.

Add the tomatoes and mix well. Stir in the chicken, mixing it with the spices. Pour in the water to cover the mixture.

Cook on medium-low heat for 20 to 30 minutes, or until the chicken is done.

YIELD: 5 to 6 servings

Chicken Souvlaki

Souvlaki is a simple Greek fast food involving marinated meat that is usually grilled. In this recipe, we made the dish on the stovetop so that you can still enjoy cooking it in the winter months. Alternatively, to grill in a more authentic atmosphere, you may move to the Greek islands.

INGREDIENTS

MARINADE

- 2 tablespoons (30 ml) lime juice
- 2 tablespoons (30 ml) olive oil
- 1/8 teaspoon salt
- 1/8 teaspoon pepper

- 2 tablespoons (30 ml) white vinegar
- 2 cloves garlic, minced
- 1/8 teaspoon ground mustard
- 1/4 teaspoon chili powder
- 1/2 teaspoon fresh sage

- 1 pound (455 g) boneless chicken breasts, cut into small pieces

To make the marinade, in a mixing bowl, combine all the marinade ingredients.

Stir in the chicken pieces and marinate for 3 to 4 hours.

Place the marinated chicken in a pan on high heat and cook until done, 10 to 15 minutes.

If you are grilling, thread the chicken pieces onto skewers and grill until cooked through, approximately 10 to 15 minutes. Remember to keep rotating the skewers so all sides cook evenly.

YIELD: 2 to 3 servings

Chicken Tagine

A tagine is a traditional Moroccan clay pot that is circular with low sides and a cone-shaped top. Unfortunately, we did not have a tagine in our kitchen, so we used a deep, ovenproof stovetop pot instead. The dish came out moist and delicious; the saffron threads add an exquisite flavor.

INGREDIENTS

MARINADE

- ¼ cup (60 ml) olive oil
- ¼ cup (15 g) fresh cilantro, chopped
- ½ teaspoon sea salt
- ¼ teaspoon saffron threads
- 2 cloves garlic, mashed
- 1 serrano chile, seeded and finely chopped

- 1 small onion, finely chopped
- ½ teaspoon cinnamon powder
- 1 teaspoon cumin powder
- ½ teaspoon powdered ginger
- ½ teaspoon turmeric powder
- ¼ teaspoon black pepper
- ¼ cup (60 ml) water

- 2 tablespoons (30 ml) olive oil
- 1 small onion, finely chopped
- 2 cloves garlic, mashed
- 1 serrano chile, seeded and finely chopped

- 1 ½ pounds (685 g) boneless chicken breasts, skinned, cleaned, and quartered
- 1/4 cup (15 g) chopped flat-leaf parsley
- 2 small Moroccan Preserved Limes, chopped (page 174)

Place the chicken pieces in a large, deep dish in a single layer. Make a few shallow knife cuts in the chicken (for marinating).

To make the marinade, combine the olive oil, cilantro, sea salt, and saffron threads in a large bowl. Mix in the garlic, chile, and chopped onion. Sprinkle in the cinnamon, cumin, ginger, turmeric, and pepper. Add the water and combine. Thoroughly coat the chicken with the marinade, working it in well. Cover the dish and marinate for at least 2 to 3 hours or overnight.

When ready to cook, preheat oven to 350°F (180°C, or gas mark 4). On the stovetop, heat the 2 tablespoons olive oil over medium heat. Add the onion, garlic, and chile. Sauté for 3 to 5 minutes. Set aside.

Place the chicken and marinade in a heavy-bottomed pot, along with the parsley, preserved limes, and stovetop mixture. If necessary, add another ¹/₄ cup (60 ml) of water to keep the mixture moist. Cook the chicken for approximately 1 hour, or until done.

YIELD: 5 to 6 servings

Zenoo's Chicken with Lemon Sauce

We were given this recipe by a member of our immediate family who has a penchant for concocting chicken-based creations that are simple but immersed in flavor. It's a nice one to have when you get home from work late on a weekday and want to make something healthy and delicious.

INGREDIENTS

- 1 pound (455 g) boneless chicken breasts
- 1 teaspoon olive oil
- $\frac{1}{2}$ teaspoon salt
- $\frac{1}{2}$ teaspoon pepper

LEMON SAUCE

- 2 tablespoons (30 ml) olive oil
- 1 small onion, minced
- 5 cloves garlic, minced
- 1 celery stick, finely chopped
- 5 mushrooms, finely chopped
- $\frac{2}{3}$ cup (155 ml) dry white wine
- $\frac{1}{4}$ cup (60 ml) lemon juice
- $\frac{1}{2}$ cup (120 ml) chicken stock (p. 47)
- 2 tablespoons (14 g) almond flour

Preheat the oven to 400°F (200°C, or gas mark 6).

To make the chicken, place the chicken breasts between two layers of waxed paper or plastic wrap and beat with a meat pounder until flattened into thin cutlets. Rub the olive oil, salt, and pepper on both sides of each cutlet, place in the oven, and cook until done, 20 to 30 minutes. Flip them over if necessary, to make sure both sides cook equally.

To make the lemon sauce, heat the olive oil in a skillet on the stovetop and sauté the minced onion and garlic for 3 to 4 minutes. Add the celery and mushrooms to the pan, and cook until soft with the cover on so you do not lose too much water. This should take 5 to 10 minutes. Pour the wine, lemon juice, and broth into the pan, and continue to cook over medium-low heat. Once the sauce starts simmering, stir in the almond flour to thicken it. Continue to simmer for another 5 to 10 minutes. Pour the sauce over the chicken and serve.

YIELD: 4 servings

NOTE: By flattening the chicken into thin cutlets, you reduce the time it needs to cook in the oven. You can also pan-sauté or grill the chicken. If you want to thicken the sauce further, add more almond flour.

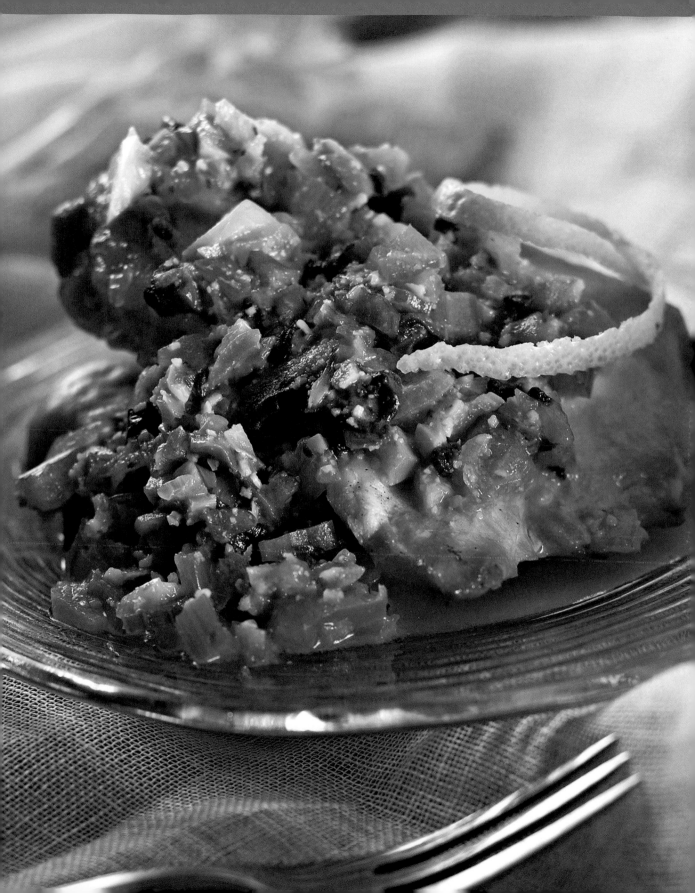

Ethiopian Chicken

The key ingredients in this recipe that give it a distinct flavor are the Ethiopian Berberé Spice (page 176) and the Spiced Butter/Ghee (page 178), both of which create a potent base from which to build the rest of the dish.

INGREDIENTS

- 2 limes, juiced
- 1 teaspoon salt, divided
- 1 1/2 pounds (685 g) boneless chicken breasts, cut into small cubes
- 2 tablespoons (28 g) Spiced Butter/Ghee (page 178) or butter
- 2 cloves garlic, finely chopped or minced
- 1 serrano chile, seeded and finely chopped
- 1 teaspoon fresh ginger, grated
- 8 spring onions, finely chopped
- 1/4 teaspoon Ethiopian Berberé Spice (page 176)
- 1 small tomato, chopped
- 1 cup (235 ml) water

In a bowl, combine the lime juice, 1/2 teaspoon of the salt, and chicken pieces. Refrigerate and allow the chicken to marinate for 1 hour.

Melt the ghee or butter in a Dutch oven or stovetop pot over medium heat. Add the garlic, chile, ginger, and spring onions, and sauté until the garlic is slightly browned, 3 to 5 minutes. Add the Berberé spice. Shake in the remaining 1/2 teaspoon salt. Stir and simmer for a few minutes. Finally, add the tomato and water. Allow everything to simmer together for 5 to 10 minutes.

Next, add the chicken pieces, making sure they are immersed in the cooking sauce. Cover the pot and simmer for 25 to 30 minutes, or until the chicken is done. Stir the chicken regularly to make sure it is cooked evenly and does not stick to the edges.

YIELD: 5 to 6 servings

Lime-Infused Chicken with Basil

Basil is an herb that has been cultivated in and around Asia for more than 5,000 years. The myths attached to basil vary according to country—as a protector against scorpions in Africa, as a transcender to God and heaven in ancient India and Egypt, and as a symbol of desire in Italy. Perhaps you can create your own myths after you sample this wonderful recipe.

INGREDIENTS

- 2 limes, juiced
- 1 cup (40 g) fresh basil leaves, finely chopped
- 3 tablespoons (45 ml) canola oil
- 1 pound (455 g) boneless and skinless chicken breasts

To make the marinade, combine the first three ingredients in a bowl.

Pierce the chicken with a fork or knife, and place it in a dish or shallow bowl. Pour the marinade over it, thoroughly coating the pieces, and let it marinate for 8 hours or overnight.

Put the marinated chicken in a stovetop pan, reserving the excess marinade, and cook over medium heat until done, 20 to 30 minutes. You don't need to add oil to the pan because there is enough oil in the marinade to prevent sticking.

Brush the chicken with the excess marinade if necessary during the cooking process.

YIELD: 2 to 3 servings

NOTE: Alternatively, you could cook the chicken on a grill.

Nonnie's Chicken and Spinach Bake

My grandmother, whom we fondly call Nonnie, made this recipe for me when I went over to her house for dinner one evening. She grew up cooking and eating primarily Italian-based recipes, and ever since I started the SCD, she has tried to adapt her recipes for me.

INGREDIENTS

- 1 ½ tablespoons (21 g) butter, divided
- 2 cloves garlic, chopped
- ¾ pound (340 g) chicken breasts, cut into bite-size pieces
- ⅓ cup (75 g) frozen spinach
- Salt and pepper to taste
- 4 ounces (115 g) Cheddar cheese

Preheat the oven to 350°F (180°C, or gas mark 4).

Heat ½ tablespoon of the butter in a saucepan, add the garlic, and cook until browned, about 2 to 3 minutes. Toss in the chicken pieces, and cook through, 15 to 20 minutes.

Meanwhile, follow the instructions on the spinach package for cooking it, either in the microwave or on the stovetop. Drain the water from the spinach.

Combine the cooked spinach with the salt, pepper, and remaining 1 tablespoon (14 g) butter, and spread the entire mixture in a small casserole dish. Place the cooked chicken on top of the spinach mixture. Slice the Cheddar cheese and lay it over the chicken.

Bake for 10 to 15 minutes, or until the cheese melts.

YIELD: 3 to 4 servings

Parmesan and Walnut Crusted Chicken

This is the SCD version of a traditional "breaded chicken" recipe, but tastier with the added walnuts and Parmesan cheese. We first discovered this recipe while visiting a close relative, who had prepared a full SCD-friendly meal for my weekend stay at her Boston home.

INGREDIENTS

- 1 pound (455 g) boneless chicken breasts
- Salt and pepper to taste
- 1 egg
- 1 tablespoon (15 ml) olive oil, divided
- 1 cup (110 g) almond flour
- 4 to 5 ounces (115 to 140 g) Parmesan cheese, grated
- 1 cup (100 g) walnuts

Preheat the oven to 375°F (190°C, or gas mark 5). Lay the chicken breasts between two sheets of waxed paper or plastic wrap. Flatten the chicken with a meat pounder until the breasts get very thin. Sprinkle salt and pepper on both sides.

Combine the egg and ½ tablespoon of the olive oil in a bowl. Put the almond flour in a separate bowl. Coat each chicken breast with the egg/olive oil mixture and then dredge both sides in the almond flour.

Coat a baking dish with the remaining 1/2 tablespoon olive oil. Place the coated chicken breasts in the baking dish. Sprinkle the Parmesan cheese on top of the chicken pieces.

Crush the walnuts into small pieces or fine crumbs. You can do this by placing the nuts in a plastic bag and breaking them with the meat pounder. Sprinkle the walnuts on top of the chicken.

Bake for 20 minutes, or until the chicken is cooked through. (You can check this by slicing the center of the fillet to see whether it is done.)

YIELD: 4 to 5 servings

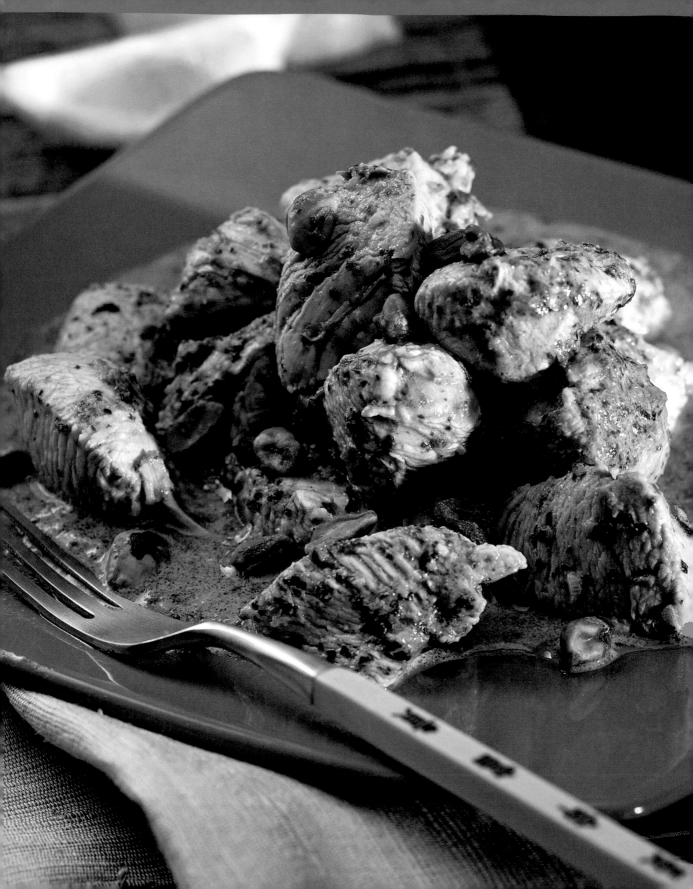

Thai Green Curry with Chicken

I would often feel a pang when we chose to order takeout from the Thai restaurant down the block from our apartment, as I scanned the menu and found only one or two SCD-friendly items. Ever since I started making this homemade Thai curry, however, the desire to get takeout has waned.

INGREDIENTS

MARINADE

- 7 to 8 spring onions, or 1 large leek, finely chopped
- 3 green chiles, seeded and finely chopped
- 2 cloves garlic, minced
- 1 tablespoon (8 g) grated fresh ginger
- 2 teaspoons coriander powder
- 1/2 teaspoon freshly ground black pepper

- 2 lemongrass stalks, trimmed and finely chopped
- 1/2 cup (20 g) fresh basil, finely chopped
- 1/2 cup (30 g) fresh cilantro, finely chopped
- 2 tablespoons (30 ml) olive oil
- 4 limes, juiced
- Salt and pepper to taste

- 1 1/2 pounds (685 g) boneless and skinless chicken breasts, diced into 1-inch (1.3-cm) cubes
- 1 tablespoon (15 ml) olive oil

- 4 ounces (115 g) SCD Coconut Milk* (page 177)
- 20 pistachio nuts

To make the marinade, combine all the marinade ingredients in a food processor until smooth. Marinate the chicken pieces in it for 1 to 2 hours in the refrigerator.

On the stovetop, heat 1 tablespoon olive oil in a stir-fry pan over medium heat. Remove the chicken pieces from the marinade, and reserve the excess marinade. Stir-fry the chicken until slightly browned, 2 to 4 minutes. Now add the reserved marinade and simmer for 3 to 5 minutes.

Next, add the coconut milk and bring to a boil. This should take 7 to 10 minutes. At this point, the chicken should be cooked through.

Garnish the dish with the pistachio nuts and serve.

YIELD: 4 to 6 servings

*NOTE: Wait at least six months after symptoms have cleared before trying coconut milk.

Sage Chicken with Portobello Mushrooms

Deemed the "humongous fungus" by some, the portobello mushroom has been used in many cultures for centuries; this delicious recipe, however, was invented fairly recently in our kitchen.

INGREDIENTS

- 1 tablespoon (15 ml) olive oil

- 5 to 6 fresh sage leaves

- 1 teaspoon salt

- 1 pound (455 g) boneless and skinless chicken breasts, diced

- 2 portobello mushroom caps, diced

Heat the olive oil in a stovetop skillet, and add the sage leaves, salt, and chicken.

Once the chicken has browned, about 5 to 7 minutes, add in the mushrooms, and cover the pan with a lid.

Allow the dish to cook until the chicken is done, approximately 10 to 15 minutes.

If there is too much water created by the mushrooms, do not cover the pan completely and allow some of the water to evaporate.

YIELD: 2 to 3 servings

Rosemary Chicken with Kalamata Olives

The olives, rosemary, and capers give this dish a distinctive Mediterranean taste—although heavy on these flavorings, it is light and smooth when done.

INGREDIENTS

- 2 tablespoons (30 ml) olive oil

- 4 cloves garlic, peeled and finely minced

- 2 1/2 pounds (1140 g) chicken breasts, whole or cut into serving pieces

- 4 sprigs fresh rosemary

- 1 1/2 cups (350 ml) dry white wine

- 5 carrots, peeled and sliced

- 2 tablespoons (17 g) SCD-safe salted capers (see chart on pages 17–18), soaked in water and drained

- 18 black kalamata olives

- Salt to taste

- 1/2 to 1 cup (120 to 235 ml) Basic Chicken or Vegetable Stock (page 46 or 47)

Heat the olive oil in a large pot. Add the garlic, chicken, and rosemary.

Sauté the chicken until it is well browned, stirring frequently, for about 10 minutes. Add the wine and stir in the carrots, capers, and olives. Add salt to taste.

Reduce heat to low, cover, and simmer for approximately 1 hour, or until the chicken is cooked through and the carrots are softened. If the mixture becomes dry, add some stock to moisten.

YIELD: 6 to 7 servings

Mom's Stuffed Chicken

This recipe blends two different stuffed chicken recipes—from both sides of our families—to come up with a new combination just for this book.

INGREDIENTS

- 1 whole chicken
- 2 tablespoons (30 ml) olive oil
- 1 teaspoon salt
- 1 teaspoon pepper
- 3 large carrots
- 8 spring onions
- 4 medium-size celery stalks
- 15 fresh sage leaves
- 10 sprigs fresh thyme
- 1/2 cup (50 g) chopped walnuts

Preheat the oven to 350°F (180°C, or gas mark 4). Grease a baking dish.

Place the chicken in the baking dish. Pierce the chicken with a fork and rub with the olive oil, salt, and pepper. Set aside.

Meanwhile, peel the carrots. Cut the carrots, spring onions, and celery into small round slices.

Mix these in a bowl with the sage, thyme, and walnuts.

Place the mixture inside the cavity of the chicken and scatter it around the dish. If possible, cut between the skin of the chicken and the meat underneath and stuff some of the mixture in between these two layers at intervals.

Bake the chicken for about 1 hour, or until cooked through.

YIELD: 4 to 6 servings

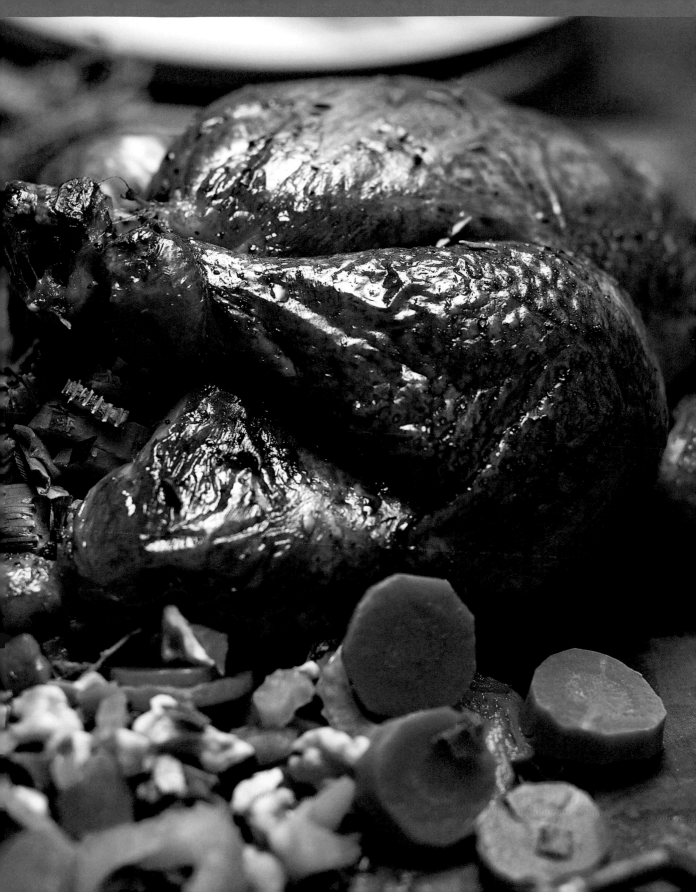

Maggie's Turkey and Prosciutto

My Aunt Maggie has a special folder in her well-organized kitchen, filled with recipe cards that she has collected over the years—handwritten, cuttings, and Xeroxed sheets. Below is one of them.

INGREDIENTS

- 1 pound (455 g) ground turkey
- 4 fresh sage leaves, finely chopped
- 6 slices SCD-safe prosciutto (see chart on pages 17–18)
- 4 tablespoons (28 g) almond flour
- Salt and pepper to taste
- 1 tablespoon (14 g) Spiced Butter/Ghee (page 178)
- 6 toothpicks

Mix together the ground turkey with the sage, so that the sage is well blended into the meat. Create 6 separate turkey cutlets, and wrap a slice of prosciutto around each one. Secure them together with a toothpick. Next, season the almond flour with salt and pepper, and dredge the turkey cutlets in the almond flour. Dust off excess flour. In a stovetop skillet, heat the ghee and sauté the cutlets on one side, until they turn brown, 5 to 10 minutes. Then remove the toothpick, and flip the cutlets over and cook the other side until done, another 5 to 10 minutes. (You can check for doneness by slicing through one of the cutlets.)

YIELD: 6 cutlets

Turkey Stir-Fry

Although turkey has its shining moment during Thanksgiving, the rest of the year it is often overlooked. We created this simple stir-fry recipe to make it part of our monthly repertoire.

INGREDIENTS

- 2 teaspoons Spiced Butter/Ghee (page 178)
- 2 cloves garlic, finely chopped
- 1 shallot, chopped
- ½ teaspoon dried cilantro flakes
- 1 teaspoon Ethiopian Berberé Spice (page 176)
- 2 cups (240 g) celeriac root
- 1 cup (120 g) grated zucchini
- 1 pound (455 g) ground turkey

Heat the ghee in a stir-fry pan, and add the garlic, shallot, salt, cilantro flakes, and Berberé spice. Cook them together for 1 to 2 minutes over medium heat. Next, add the grated turnips, zucchini, and ground turkey. Stir-fry until the turkey is done, 10 to 15 minutes.

YIELD: 4 to 5 servings

CHAPTER 9

Seafood

When we lived in Brooklyn, we bought a 15-inch-long fish in Chinatown, and traveled back with it iced, determined to grill it.

My mother is the family fishing expert, the one who used to have us wade out with nets to catch bait before going blue snapper fishing, the one who always caught fish, and the one who could clean a fish so fast that it stunned my dad's war veteran friends. So I telephoned her for instructions. However, before she could explain, an urgent call came on the other line. While I stayed on the phone, my wife Nilou went ahead and cleaned the fish.

During phone calls I tend to pace, so as I reached the end of the kitchen section of our cozy apartment, I glanced at Nilou. Scales were all over the wall above the cutting board. Each time I walked over, the fish had become smaller and smaller. By the end of the phone call, the fish had gone from 15 inches to three small, shredded clumps. There wasn't much left to cook.

Determined, we started up the tiny charcoal grill that sat on our fire escape, and put the fish pieces on, without foil. Within minutes, they shrunk and slid through the grating into the fire. Laughing at our culinary disaster, we went back inside and ordered takeout.

Over the past six years, our cooking of fish has greatly improved now—thanks in part to plenty of advice from my mother—though now we almost always buy fillets or have the whole fish cleaned at the local market.

Aunt Jo's Mussels

Growing up, my mom's relatives held an annual summer family picnic. Everyone came for the daylong event to play pinochle and bocce, go swimming, and reconnect. During dinner, a giant pot of mussels was bought out for everyone to dig into. Thanks to Aunt Jo and Cousin Jeanette, we now have this delicious recipe in our book.

INGREDIENTS

- 3 pounds (1365 g) mussels or clams, or a combination of both, washed
- 1/4 cup (60 ml) water
- 2 tablespoons (8 g) fresh parsley, finely chopped
- 1 tablespoon (10 g) minced garlic
- 2 teaspoons salt
- 1 teaspoon oregano
- 1/4 cup (60 ml) vegetable or olive oil
- Pinch of red pepper flakes
- Melted butter, for serving (optional)

Place the mussels in a large, deep pot. Add the remaining ingredients (except for the butter), cover, and cook on medium-high until the mixture begins to boil.

Lower the heat to medium and simmer until the mussels open, approximately 3 to 5 minutes. Discard any that fail to open. Serve immediately with melted butter, if desired.

YIELD: 2 to 3 servings

NOTE: Check the mussels when washing them. If a mussel is open, tap it lightly. If the shell doesn't close, discard it. Also discard any that do not open after cooking.

Spicy Shrimp with Mustard Seeds

Mustard seeds have been around for eons—they are mentioned in both ancient Sanskrit writings and Greek medicine. They are the seeds of the mustard plant. This dish is great as an appetizer for a small dinner party, but it can also be made for a main course.

INGREDIENTS

- 2 cloves garlic, mashed
- 1-inch (2.5-cm) piece fresh ginger, peeled and grated
- 1 teaspoon turmeric powder
- 1 teaspoon chili powder
- 2 teaspoons whole black mustard seeds*
- 1/4 teaspoon cardamom powder
- 2 tablespoons (28 g) butter, divided
- 1 pound (455 g) shrimp, cleaned and deveined, with tails attached
- 1/4 cup (60 ml) SCD Coconut Milk* (page 177)
- Salt and pepper to taste
- Fresh cilantro, chopped, for garnish

In a bowl, combine the garlic, ginger, turmeric, chili powder, mustard seeds, and cardamom powder. In a separate bowl, place the shrimp.

In a small pan, melt 1 tablespoon (14 g) of the butter. Add the spice mixture and stir until thoroughly incorporated, about 1 to 2 minutes. Remove from heat and add the mixture to the shrimp, coating thoroughly. Cover and marinate for 1 hour in the refrigerator.

Melt the remaining 1 tablespoon (14 g) butter in a stovetop sauté pan over medium heat. Add the shrimp and cook, stirring continuously, for 3 to 5 minutes. Add the coconut milk, salt, and pepper, and simmer for 5 to 8 minutes. The shrimp should be opaque when done. Garnish the dish with the cilantro.

YIELD: 3 to 4 servings

NOTE: You can find black mustard seeds at most Asian grocery stores.

*NOTE: Wait at least three months after symptoms have cleared before trying seeds. Wait at least six months after symptoms have cleared before trying coconut milk.

Herbed Tilapia with Lime

This type of fish is very soft, and does not require too much fuss. We came up with this recipe because we had two fillets of tilapia that needed to be cooked immediately. The preparation time was not more than 5 minutes, and the cooking time was 10 to 15 minutes.

INGREDIENTS

- 1 tablespoon (15 ml) olive oil
- 1/8 teaspoon thyme
- 1/8 teaspoon dried basil
- 1/4 teaspoon salt
- 3/4 pound (340 g) tilapia fillets
- 1/2 lime, juiced

Heat the olive oil over medium heat in a stovetop pan. Sprinkle the thyme, basil, and salt equally on both sides of the fillets. Add the fillets to the pan.

Cook the fish for 10 to 15 minutes, or until cooked through. Place on serving plates, sprinkle the lime juice over the fillets, and serve.

YIELD: 2 servings

NOTE: Mango Salsa (page 94) would be a great side for this recipe.

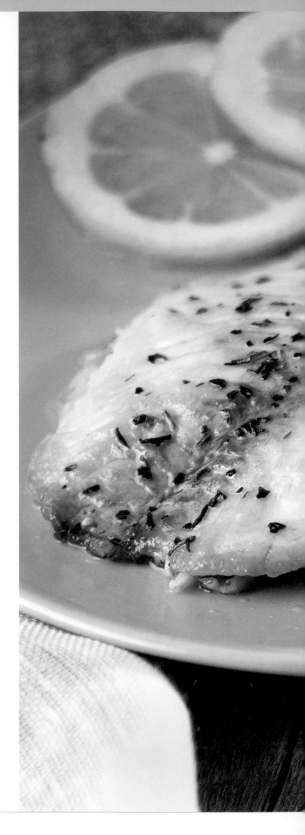

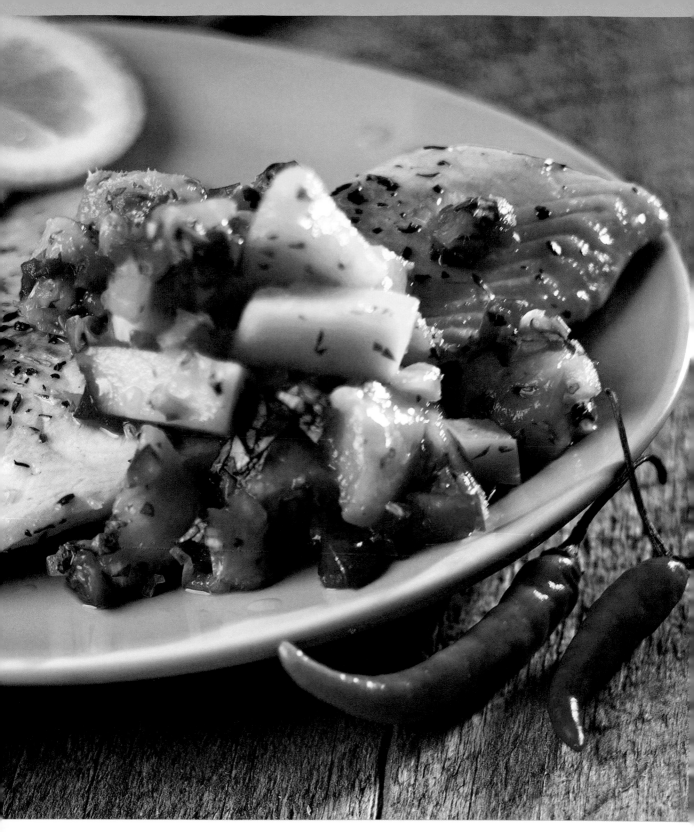

Cameroon Peanut Fish

The preparation of fish for this Central African recipe does not require it to be cooked as a fillet, but more as a shredded version that is tossed together with the other ingredients in the peanut sauce.

INGREDIENTS

- 1 tablespoon (15 ml) peanut oil
- 5 cloves garlic, minced
- 2 serrano chiles, seeded and finely chopped
- 2 small onions, finely chopped
- 1/2 teaspoon coriander powder
- 1/2 teaspoon ground nutmeg powder
- 1/2 teaspoon salt
- 1/2 teaspoon black pepper
- 1 1/4 pounds (570 g) tilapia fillets, chopped into bite-size pieces
- 3/4 cup (195 g) SCD-safe peanut butter (see chart on pages 17–18)
- 3/4 cup (175 ml) warm water
- 3 sprigs cilantro, for garnish

Heat the peanut oil in a wok or stir-fry pan over medium heat. Sauté the garlic, chiles, and onions for 3 to 4 minutes, until lightly browned. Add the coriander, nutmeg, salt, pepper, and fish and cook until the fish is done, about 10 to 15 minutes.

Meanwhile, in a separate bowl, combine the peanut butter and water until the peanut butter is diluted into the water and softened. This will allow the peanut butter flavor to be infused more easily into the fish. Add this mixture to the pan, and stir-fry for about 1 minute until the mixture is evenly distributed. Garnish with the cilantro before serving.

YIELD: 6 to 8 servings

Glazed Salmon with Ginger

Folklore, and consequent research, has shown that salmon always go back to their own birthplaces to create the next generation. When I went to Alaska seeking summer adventure as a young college student, I did not realize the amount of salmon I would be surrounded by—always a constant staple among the unique characters and moments I experienced there. In more recent years, I have come to appreciate the strong flavor of this fish.

INGREDIENTS

- 3-inch (7.5-cm) piece fresh ginger
- 2 cloves garlic
- 6 tablespoons (90 ml) SCD Asian Sauce (page 173)
- 1 teaspoon sesame oil
- 1 tablespoon (20 g) honey
- 1 ½ pounds (685 g) wild salmon, cut into 3 or 4 fillets
- Sesame seeds,* for garnish (optional)

Peel the ginger and garlic, grate them, and place them in a bowl.

Add the sauce, sesame oil, and honey to the bowl, and whisk all the ingredients together until thoroughly mixed. Marinate the fish in the sauce for 30 to 45 minutes.

Preheat the oven to 325°F (170°C or gas mark 3). Oil an ovenproof baking dish, and lay the fish in the pan, skin side down. Reserve the excess marinade. Bake for 7 to 10 minutes without turning, basting frequently with the excess marinade. Check the doneness of the fish by testing with a fork—the fish should easily flake apart.

Garnish with sesame seeds, if desired. To prepare the sesame seeds, dry-roast them in a small skillet on the stovetop until they just turn light brown (less than a minute), and then sprinkle them on top of the salmon fillets.

YIELD: 3 to 4 servings

*NOTE: Wait at least three months after symptoms have cleared before trying seeds.

Zenobia's Wild Salmon over Vegetables

This fish dish is unusual in that we use one large fillet piece, and soak it in the flavors from the cooked vegetables underneath.

INGREDIENTS

- 1 1/2 pounds (685 g) wild salmon, skinned
- Salt and pepper to taste
- 1 tablespoon (15 ml) sesame oil
- 3/4 tablespoon olive oil
- 3 cloves garlic, minced
- 1 large onion, finely chopped
- 2 medium-size zucchini, finely chopped
- 3 to 4 portobello mushroom caps, finely chopped

Preheat the oven to 350°F (180°C, or gas mark 4). Lightly coat a baking dish with oil and set aside.

Place the salmon between two sheets of waxed paper or plastic wrap and flatten it with a meat pounder until thin. Rub salt and pepper on the fillet. Coat the top with the sesame oil. Set aside.

Heat the olive oil in a pan on the stovetop and sauté the garlic and onion for 3 to 5 minutes over medium heat. Add the zucchini and mushrooms, cover, and cook for approximately 20 minutes.

Place the vegetable mixture in the baking dish, and then put the flattened salmon on top (skin side down). Bake for 15 to 20 minutes. The salmon cooks faster than usual not only because of its thinness, but also because the heat from the vegetables speeds up the process.

YIELD: 7 to 8 servings

Nafisa's Spicy Fried Fish

One of the fresh fish markets in Mumbai (formerly Bombay), India, can be found by winding your way through a crowded, nondescript gulley near Grant Road Station. It is set in an old Victorian building, a colonial remnant with 30-foot-high ceilings and ancient fans droning above. The hustle and bustle of the machhiwalis (fisherwomen), luring customers to buy their freshly caught merchandise, greets you as you first enter. The machhiwalis are decked out in their finest jewelry (they wear their earnings on themselves) and laugh merrily—their cutting knives sparkling as much as the jewelry they wear.

INGREDIENTS

- 1 tablespoon (15 ml) freshly squeezed lime juice
- ¼ teaspoon red chili powder
- ¼ teaspoon turmeric powder
- ½ teaspoon salt
- 1 pound (455 g) firm fish fillets,* such as sole, halibut, or bass
- 2 tablespoons (30 ml) olive oil
- Lime wedges, for garnish

Combine the lime juice, chili powder, turmeric, and salt in a bowl large enough to hold the fillets. Marinate the fish in the mixture for half an hour.

Heat the olive oil in a stovetop pan over medium-high heat. Place the fish fillets in the pan and cook until the bottom is done, 4 to 5 minutes,

Turn over and cook for at least 3 more minutes. Let cook until the fillets reach a crisp consistency and the fish is firm.

Garnish with lime wedges and serve.

YIELD: 3 to 4 servings

*__NOTE:__ Use a fish that is good for frying, so it will hold together and not fall apart.

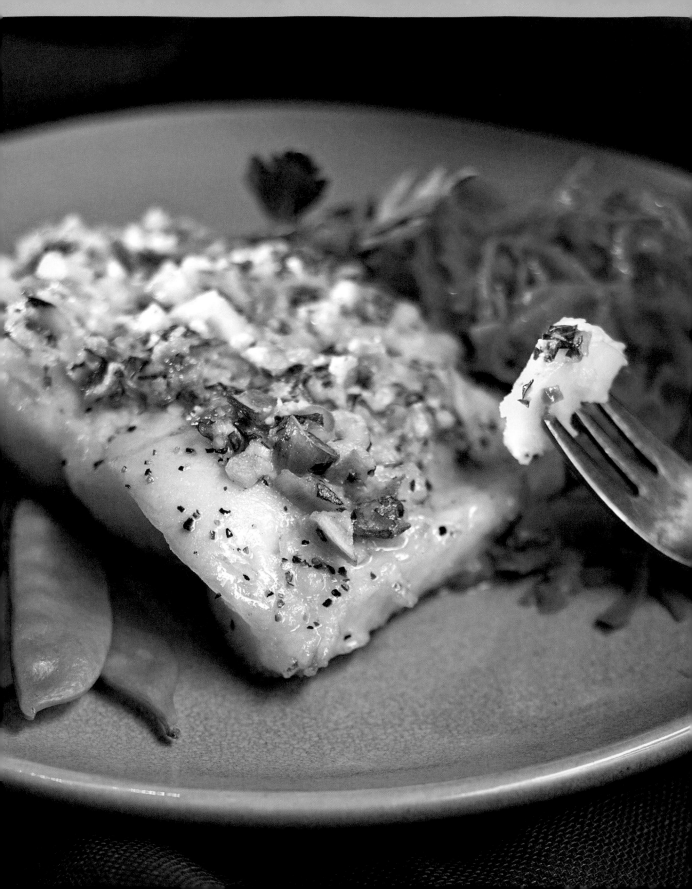

Roasted Bass with Parsley Butter

Picture a dark brown table with matching chairs, nicely laid out with table settings for four people. Conversation is flowing, classical music is playing, and a warm breeze is softly billowing the sheer white curtains hanging on the windows. After the initial wine and appetizers, the main entree is brought out. This quick and succulent fish dish is great for small, sit-down dinner parties like this one.

INGREDIENTS

BUTTER

- 4 tablespoons (55 g) butter, softened
- 1 ½ tablespoons (10 g) almond flour
- 2 shallots, minced
- 1 clove garlic, mashed

- 4 tablespoons (16 g) chopped parsley
- 3 limes, juiced
- Salt and pepper to taste

- 1 tablespoon (15 ml) olive oil
- 4 fillets of bass, sole, halibut, or any other firm whitefish
- Salt and pepper to taste

For the butter, thoroughly combine the almond flour, shallots, garlic, parsley, lime juice, and softened butter in a bowl. Add salt and pepper to taste. The butter can be made in advance and stored in the refrigerator wrapped in plastic wrap. Before using, make sure it is softened.

Preheat the oven to 400°F (200°C, or gas mark 6).

Heat the oil in a skillet over medium heat. Season the fish with salt and pepper and then add to the pan, skin side down, and cook until golden brown, about 5 minutes. Turn the fish over and cook for 2 more minutes. Remove the fillets from the pan and place them in an ovenproof dish (the less cooked side facing up). Spoon a tablespoon of the butter over each fillet and roast in the oven for 10 minutes.

To serve, place each fillet on a plate and drizzle the remaining butter over the fish.

YIELD: 4 servings

NOTE: You can also use this butter over grilled vegetables or shrimp.

Traditional Christmas Fish

Christmas every year means at least one fish entrée on the formal dining table. This recipe has become part of our holiday tradition for the past few years.

INGREDIENTS

- Toothpicks, one for each fillet
- 3/4 pound (340 g) sole fillets
- 4 tablespoons (55 g) butter, melted
- 1/2 cup plus 2 tablespoons (60 g) grated Parmesan cheese, divided
- 2 cloves garlic, minced
- 1 teaspoon grated lime zest
- 1 1/2 teaspoons dried dill
- 1/4 teaspoon salt
- 1/2 teaspoon pepper
- 1 carrot, peeled and cut into small pieces
- 1 celery stalk, cut into small pieces
- 1/4 teaspoon paprika

Place toothpicks in a bowl of water and let soak. This prevents them from burning in the oven. Preheat the oven to 375°F (190°C, or gas mark 5). Butter a baking dish.

Pat the fillets dry and spread them on a baking sheet.

Combine the butter, 1/2 cup (50 g) of the Parmesan cheese, garlic, lime zest, dill, salt, pepper, carrot, and celery in a bowl. Divide the mixture into equal size portions for as many fillets as you have. Spread the mixture across each fillet, roll the fillet, and secure with a toothpick.

Place the fillets, rolled sides down, in the baking dish. Sprinkle the tops of each fillet with paprika and the remaining 2 tablespoons (10 g) Parmesan cheese. Bake on the top rack for 30 minutes.

When done, turn the oven to broil and place the fish under the broiler for 2 to 3 minutes to brown the tops.

YIELD: 3 to 4 servings

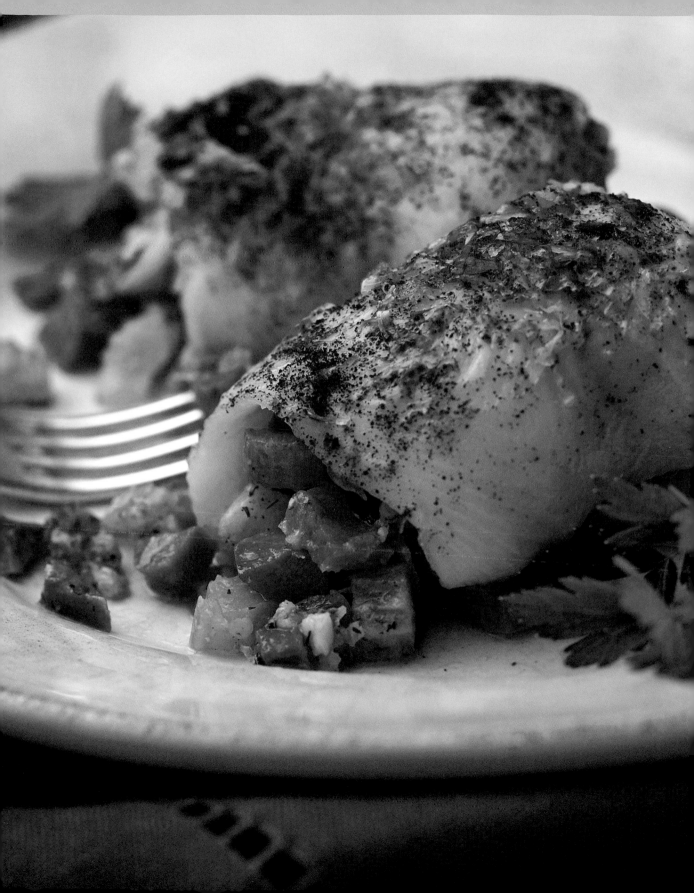

Sophie's Trout with Pesto Sauce

The lightness of this pan-fried fish and the heaviness of the pesto blend together nicely to stimulate the senses.

INGREDIENTS

PESTO

- 2 cups (80 g) packed fresh basil leaves
- 1/3 cup (45 g) pine nuts
- 3 cloves garlic, minced
- 1/2 cup (120 ml) extra virgin olive oil
- 1/2 cup (50 g) freshly grated Parmesan cheese
- Salt and freshly ground black pepper to taste

FISH

- 3 tablespoons (45 ml) olive oil
- 2 1/4 pounds (1025 g) trout
- 2 limes, juiced
- 1 tablespoon (3 g) basil, finely chopped
- 1 tablespoon (9 g) pine nuts
- 4 limes, halved

To make the pesto, combine the basil and pine nuts in a food processor or blender. Pulse a few times. Add the garlic and pulse some more. Slowly add the olive oil into the chute while the food processor is running. Keep stopping to scrape the sides of the food processor with a spatula. Add the cheese and blend again until the consistency becomes smooth. Add a little salt and freshly ground black pepper to taste.

For the fish, heat the 3 tablespoons (45 ml) olive oil in a large pan. Add the trout and pour the lime juice over it. Pan-fry the trout for 4 minutes on each side. Add the basil and pine nuts and cook for an additional 2 to 3 minutes. Remove from the pan and set aside.

To serve, place a spoonful of pesto on top of each piece of trout. Serve with the lime halves.

YIELD: 4 to 6 servings

NOTE: Instead of pan-frying the trout, you can rub the fish with salt, pepper, and olive oil, and then grill it. To serve, simply heap a spoonful of the pesto on top of each fillet.

CHAPTER 10

Meat

In the corner of my Aunt Maggie's house stands a worn but solid block of wood on four short legs. The edges of the block are smooth to the touch and the top slopes and ripples. The butcher's block hasn't been used for decades, but it was once part of my grandparents' store in New Haven, Connecticut.

After returning from World War II, my grandfather, George Swanson, started a small store that sold meat, canned goods, and a few vegetables. One of the first purchases for the store was the butcher's block. The block followed them when they moved down the street to a larger space and began carrying a wider selection of groceries, as well as a memorable counter of assorted penny candy. When not making deliveries, Grandpa George spent much of his time wearing his apron, standing behind the butcher's block, and sharpening his knives to prepare orders.

Sunday mornings were some of the busiest. At 5:30 a.m., he would go to the bakery to buy bags of crusty, seeded loaves and rolls. By 6:30 a.m. my mother and grandmother had lined up the bags, identified by customers' names, and filled them with their orders. By the time church let out, they would be ready for the morning rush. People picked up the bags, ordered deli meats, and walked around the store to buy a few more items.

Although she's too humble to say such a thing, my grandmother was well known in the neighborhood for her cooking. My aunt tells of many newly married women coming to the store, not only to buy food, but also to ask her advice on certain dishes. Also, in the summers, boaters on the Quinnipiac River would pull ashore and walk the few blocks to the store. They'd buy sandwiches made of Italian bread, layered with cold cuts, lettuce, and tomato, and then add a side of something my grandmother had prepared that morning: potato salad, macaroni salad, or coleslaw.

My grandfather died before I was born. In most families, heirlooms are often passed down through the generations. The same is true for our family, except one item is larger than average: the butcher block, which my aunt has preserved to help keep alive memories of my grandparents and their store.

Beef and Broccoli, Chinese-Style

This recipe uses flavorful sesame oil as a substitute for non-SCD-safe soy and other sauces that are often used in Chinese cooking. The toasted sesame seed and oil base enhances the stir-fry by imparting a delicious Asian flavor to the dish.

INGREDIENTS

- 1 to 1 1/2 pounds (455 to 685 g) broccoli florets (6 to 9 cups [420 to 630 g])
- 1 1/4 pounds (570 g) eye of round beef steak
- 2 tablespoons (30 ml) sesame oil, divided
- 10 cloves garlic, finely chopped
- 1/2 teaspoon salt
- 1/2 teaspoon white pepper
- 1 teaspoon sesame seeds*

Cut the broccoli into bite-size florets. Place in a steamer and steam until desired tenderness is reached, or about 7 to 10 minutes. Set aside.

Trim the excess fat from the beef, and cut into small pieces, approximately 1 inch (2.5 cm) in length and 1/8 to 1/4 inch (3 to 6 mm) in width.

In a wok, over medium heat, heat 1 tablespoon (15 ml) of the oil and sauté the garlic until browned, 3 to 5 minutes. Add the beef, salt, and white pepper, and toss together. Cook until the beef is almost cooked through, 15 to 20 minutes. Turn the heat to high, and add the broccoli and 3/4 tablespoon of the sesame oil to the wok, stir-frying for 1 to 2 minutes, or until the beef is done.

Just before you are ready to serve the dish, heat the remaining 1/4 tablespoon sesame oil in a small pan and roast the sesame seeds until golden, less than 1 minute. Do not allow them to overcook or they will burn. Add to the stir-fry and toss to combine.

YIELD: 4 to 6 servings

*NOTE: Wait at least three months after symptoms have cleared before trying seeds.

Beef Vindaloo

Centuries ago, Vindaloo was bought to India by the Portuguese, specifically to the coastal area where Goa is located—a place known for its beaches and slower pace of life. This dish integrates the local versions we tasted during our visits there. We adjusted this version to be less spicy than the traditional Vindaloo.

INGREDIENTS

- 2 tablespoons (28 g) butter or Spiced Butter/Ghee (page 178)
- 1 large onion
- 2 cloves garlic
- 2 tablespoons (30 ml) red wine vinegar
- 1 teaspoon honey
- 1/2 cup (120 ml) water
- 2 medium-size tomatoes, diced
- 1 1/4 pounds (570 g) rib-eye beef, chopped into 1-inch (2.5-cm) cubes
- 1/2 cup (30 g) fresh cilantro, chopped

VINDALOO SPICE MIXTURE

- 1 teaspoon coriander powder
- 2 teaspoons cumin powder
- 1-inch (2.5-cm) piece ginger, peeled and finely minced
- 1 cinnamon stick
- 2 bay leaves
- 4 whole cloves
- 1/4 teaspoon chili powder
- 1/8 teaspoon cardamom powder
- 1/8 teaspoon turmeric powder
- 1/4 teaspoon black pepper
- 1/2 teaspoon salt
- 1 whole star anise

In a large stovetop pan, heat the butter or ghee and sauté the onions and garlic for 3 to 4 minutes, or until tender.

To make the spice mixture, combine all the ingredients in a small bowl. Add the mixture to the onions and garlic. Immediately stir in the vinegar, honey, water, and tomatoes. Bring to a boil.

Add the beef and bring to a boil again. Reduce the heat, cover, and simmer for 1 hour, stirring occasionally.

Remove the cover and simmer until the liquid is reduced by half, 15 to 20 minutes.

Top with the fresh cilantro and serve.

YIELD: 4 to 6 servings

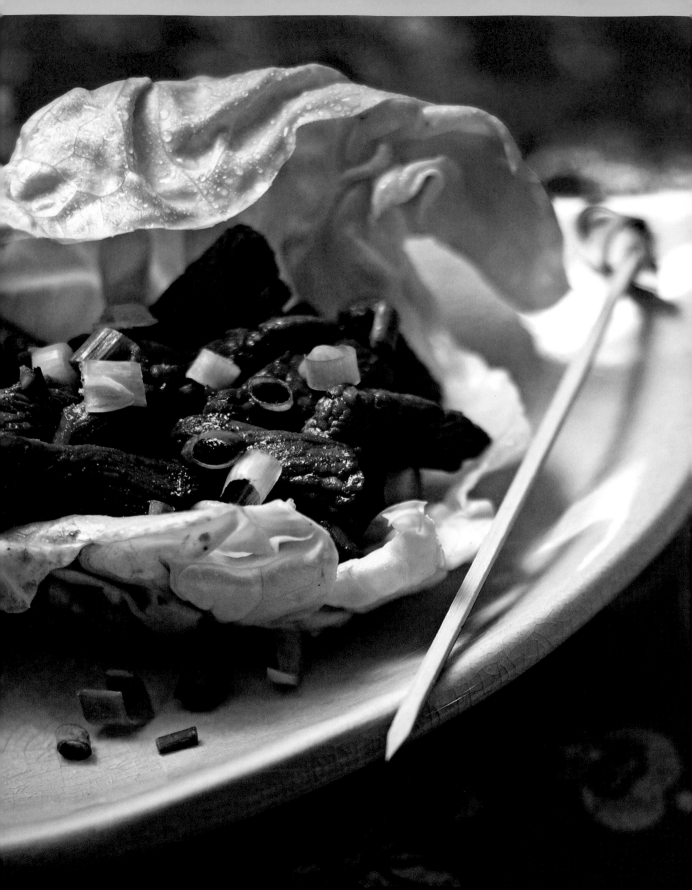

Bulgogi Wraps
(Korean Marinated Beef)

Bulgogi literally translates as "fire meat" in Korean cuisine, and it is one of the most popular dishes in Korea. The meat is traditionally grilled over a flame, but pan-cooking can be used as an alternative—as in this recipe, where we have chosen to pan-fry it on top of the stove.

INGREDIENTS

- 1 pound (455 g) rib-eye beef
- $\frac{1}{4}$ cup (60 ml) SCD Asian Sauce (page 173)
- $\frac{1}{3}$ cup (80 ml) sesame oil
- 2 tablespoons (40 g) honey
- 3 cloves garlic, finely chopped
- 8 to 10 spring onions, finely chopped
- Pepper and salt to taste
- 5 to 6 lettuce leaves

Cut the beef into thin slices. Set aside.

Combine the remaining ingredients, except the lettuce, in a large bowl. Add the beef, and marinate for 1 hour.

Stir-fry the beef on top of the stove over medium-high heat until it is cooked through, 10 to 15 minutes.

Wash the lettuce leaves, and place alongside the beef. Wrap the leaf around the beef, and eat!

YIELD: 2 to 3 servings

Mom's Chili Beef

This recipe needs special attention because of the required presoaking of the red kidney beans, but it is well worth the extra effort.

INGREDIENTS

- ⅓ cup (65 g) dried red kidney beans*
- 1 tablespoon (15 ml) olive oil
- 2 cloves garlic, chopped
- 1 medium-size onion, chopped
- 1 tablespoon (5 g) chili powder

- 1 teaspoon cumin powder
- 1 pound (455 g) ground beef
- 1 green bell pepper, cored and diced
- 5 plum tomatoes, chopped

Soak the kidney beans in water for 10 to 14 hours—the water level should be above the beans. During this time, rinse the beans and add fresh water if the water becomes too bubbly from the "gas" released from the beans.

After soaking, cook the beans by putting them in a pot of fresh water, bringing the water to a boil, and then simmering until they are soft and cooked through, 1 to 2 hours.

In a separate stovetop pan, heat the olive oil, and brown the garlic and onion for 2 to 4 minutes. Add the chili and cumin powders, and stir for 1 to 2 minutes. Add the beef, bell pepper, and tomatoes, and cook until done, approximately 20 minutes. Add the pre-cooked, drained kidney beans and mix until well blended.

YIELD: 8 to 10 servings

*NOTE: Wait at least three months after symptoms have cleared before trying beans. Do not use canned beans.

"Pasta-less" Lasagna

This lasagna variation uses spaghetti squash, tomato sauce, and ground beef.
Many of the parts are cooked separately and then assembled together at the end.

INGREDIENTS

- 1 1/2 teaspoons olive oil, divided
- 1 medium-size onion, diced
- 4 cloves garlic, minced
- 1 pound (455 g) ground beef
- 1 teaspoon salt
- 1 teaspoon dried oregano

- 1 teaspoon dried basil
- 1 spaghetti squash, peeled, seeded, and chopped into pieces
- 1 1/2 cups (350 ml) Mom's Tomato Sauce (page 172)
- 1 1/2 cups (150 g) grated Cheddar cheese

Preheat the oven to 350°F (180°C, or gas mark 4).

Heat 1 teaspoon of the olive oil in a skillet over medium heat and cook the onion and garlic for 2 to 4 minutes. Add the beef, salt, oregano, and basil. Stir well, and sauté until the beef is cooked through, 10 to 15 minutes.

Meanwhile, steam the spaghetti squash pieces until soft (but not too soft). They will be done when a fork can pierce them, and they come out "stringy." Place the steamed pieces in a mixing bowl, and whisk with a fork for 1 minute to make sure the "chunks" loosen into thin, spaghetti-like strands. Set aside.

Grease the bottom of a baking pan or casserole dish with the remaining ½ teaspoon olive oil, and spread out half the steamed spaghetti squash. Pour half of the tomato sauce over the squash. Next, add a layer of half of the ground beef over the sauce. Sprinkle half of the cheese over the beef. Repeat the process again, using up the remaining squash, sauce, beef, and cheese, ending with a layer of cheese.

Bake in the oven for 5 to 10 minutes, or until the cheese melts.

YIELD: 8 to 10 servings

NOTE: To make this dish vegetarian, omit the beef.

Moroccan Beef with Spices

"Of all the gin joints in all the towns in all the world, she walks into mine."
If you are a romantic at heart, you may remember the silver screen lines mut-
tered by the cigarette-puffing Humphrey Bogart when Ingrid Bergman makes
her appearance in the movie Casablanca. *Bogart and Bergman aside, tradi-*
tional Moroccan food has always been a cross-cultural mix of influences from
parts of Africa, the Middle East, and Mediterranean Europe, centuries before
Casablanca *was scripted. We borrowed this recipe from a friend and modified*
it for the SCD.

INGREDIENTS

MARINADE

- 1 medium-size onion, grated or finely chopped
- 1/2 cup (30 g) chopped fresh parsley
- 3 cloves garlic, finely minced
- 2 tablespoons (30 g) SCD Yogurt (page 19)
- 1 teaspoon cumin powder
- 1/4 teaspoon cayenne pepper
- 1/16 teaspoon cardamom powder
- 1/8 teaspoon cinnamon powder
- 1/8 teaspoon clove powder
- Salt and pepper to taste
- 2 tablespoons (30 ml) olive oil

- 1 1/2 pounds (350 g) steak fillets, about 1 inch (2.5 cm) thick and trimmed of excess fat

To make the marinade, combine the marinade ingredients in a bowl. Spread the marinade thickly over each side of the steak filets. Cover and refrigerate overnight, or for a minimum of 3 hours.

Cook the marinated steaks on a grill until they've reached the desired doneness, 20 to 30 minutes.

YIELD: 6 to 8 servings

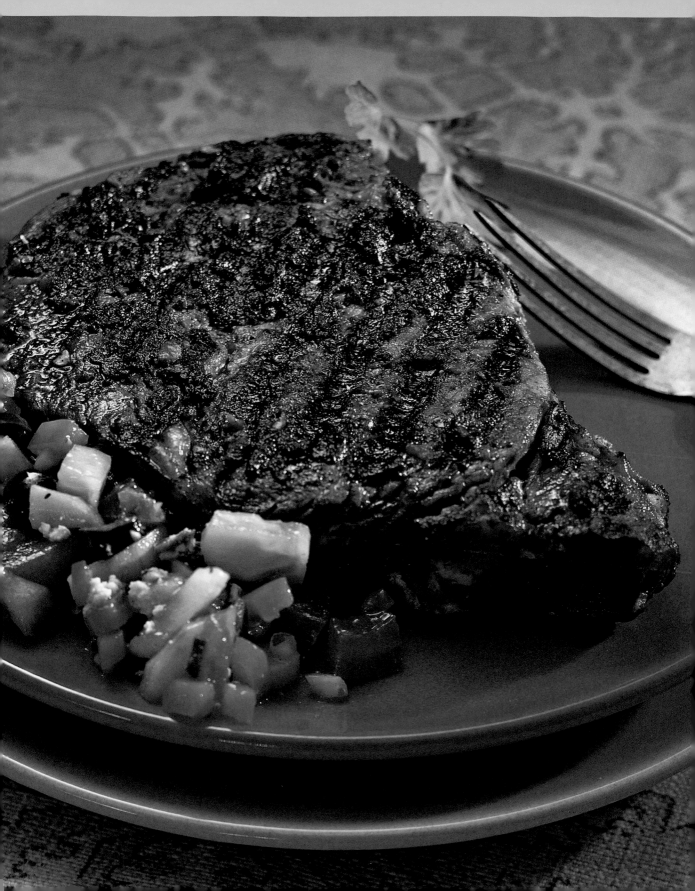

Perfect London Roast

This roast is effortless to prepare—you only need 5 to 10 minutes of prep work before putting it into the oven. Enjoy it with a nice glass of red wine!

INGREDIENTS

- 7 cloves garlic, finely minced
- 1 tablespoon (15 ml) olive oil
- 1 teaspoon salt
- 1 teaspoon black pepper
- 1 ¼ pounds (570 g) sirloin steak

Preheat the oven to 350°F (180°C, or gas mark 4). Mix together the garlic, olive oil, salt, and black pepper. Rub the mixture on the steak.

Place the steak in a baking dish and cook for 30 to 40 minutes, or until the desired doneness is reached.

YIELD: 2 to 3 servings

Ruma's Layered Pot Roast

A friend of the family, Ruma, gave us this recipe many years ago. The slow cooking of the beef is the key to releasing the rich, juicy flavors of this dish.

INGREDIENTS

- 1 large onion, finely chopped
- 1 clove garlic, finely chopped
- 1 tablespoon (9 g) SCD-safe capers (see chart on pages 17–18), chopped
- ¼ cup (15 g) fresh parsley, chopped
- 3 tablespoons (45 ml) olive oil, divided
- 1 pound (455 g) boneless beef, cut into thin slices

Combine the onion, garlic, capers, and parsley in a bowl. Set aside.

Pour 2 tablespoons (30 ml) of the olive oil into a stovetop pot. Arrange a layer of meat slices in the pot and spread the onion mixture on top. Keep alternating beef and onion layers, finishing with a layer of the onion mixture. Pour the remaining 1 tablespoon (15 ml) olive oil on top of the last layer, and cover the pot with a lid.

Cook at a bare simmer, over low heat, until the meat is tender, about 1 hour.

YIELD: 4 to 5 servings

Yunus's Kheema

This dish was my father-in-law's speciality during his bachelor days. He still makes it during his visits to the U.S., when we put him to work in the kitchen.

INGREDIENTS

- 1 tablespoon (15 ml) olive oil
- 1 onion, chopped
- 2 cloves garlic, minced
- 1 jalapeño chile pepper, seeded and diced
- 2 whole cloves
- 1 cinnamon stick
- 1/2 teaspoon peeled and grated ginger

- 1/2 teaspoon coriander powder
- 1/2 teaspoon turmeric powder
- 1/2 teaspoon cumin powder
- Salt to taste
- 1 pound (455 g) ground beef
- 2 small tomatoes, diced
- 1/3 cup (20 g) fresh cilantro, chopped

In a saucepan, heat the olive oil over medium heat and sauté the onion and garlic for 2 to 3 minutes. Add the jalapeño pepper and all the spices and cook together for 1 to 2 minutes. Next, mix in the beef, tomatoes, and cilantro. Cook together for 15 to 20 minutes, or until the beef is cooked through. Remove the whole cloves and cinnamon stick before serving.

YIELD: 3 to 4 servings

Frikadellen (German Hamburgers)

This German version of the hamburger dates back to seventeenth-century Europe. In the variation below, we decided to use almond flour instead of bread.

INGREDIENTS

- 1 Vidalia onion, finely chopped
- 3 tablespoons (21 g) almond flour
- 1 pound (455 g) ground beef
- 1 egg

- Salt and pepper to taste
- 1/2 teaspoon fresh thyme
- 2 cloves garlic, minced
- 1 tablespoon (15 ml) olive oil

Combine all the ingredients (except the olive oil) in a bowl and mix well. Form meat patties and set aside.

Heat the olive oil in a stovetop pan and sauté the patties on both sides until cooked through, approximately 7 minutes for each side.

YIELD: 6 to 8 servings

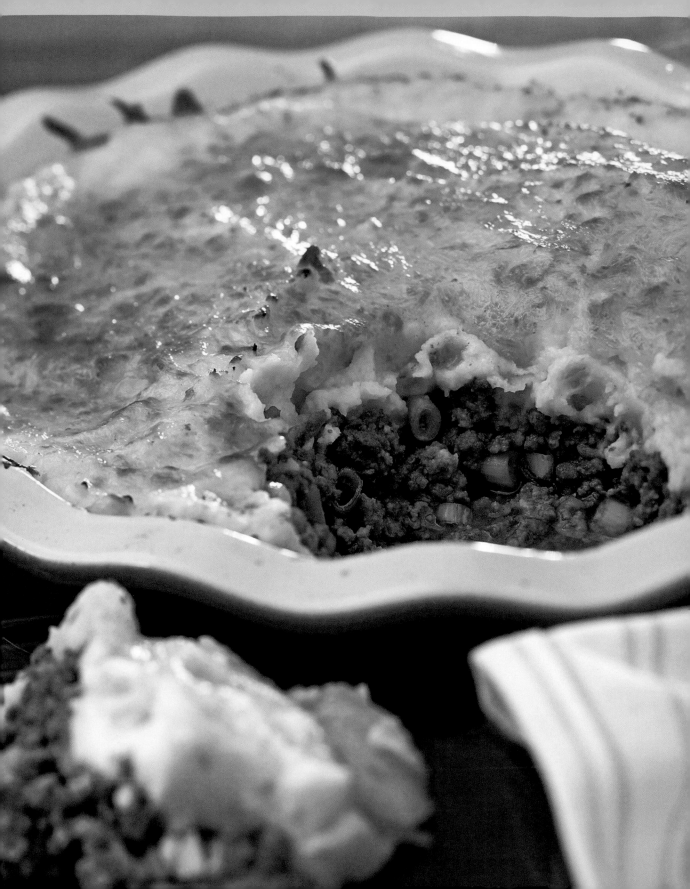

Shepherd's Pie

This recipe is a two-step process, which, when combined, tastes delicious! It is an attempt to create a traditional English dish without the traditional English ingredients.

INGREDIENTS

- 1 1/2 tablespoons (23 ml) olive oil, divided
- 1 pound (455 g) ground beef
- 1/2 teaspoon cumin powder
- 1 teaspoon salt
- 1/2 teaspoon pepper
- 10 spring onions, finely chopped
- 2 tablespoons (30 ml) lime juice
- 1 medium-size cauliflower, cut into florets
- 2 tablespoons (28 g) butter
- 3/4 cup (90 g) grated Cheddar cheese
- Parsley leaves, for garnish (optional)

Preheat the oven to 325°F (170°C, or gas mark 3). Grease an ovenproof baking dish with 1/2 tablespoon (8 ml) of the olive oil.

In a stovetop pan, heat the remaining 1 tablespoon (15 ml) olive oil and sauté the ground beef for 1 to 2 minutes.

Add the cumin powder, salt, and pepper and cook over low heat until the ground beef is cooked through, another 15 to 20 minutes.

Add the spring onions to the mixture and stir for about 2 minutes, or until they soften slightly. Remove the pan from the stove, and mix in the lime juice. Place the mixture in the ovenproof baking dish.

Meanwhile, steam the cauliflower florets until tender. Purée or blend the cauliflower with the butter in a food processor until smooth. Then spread it evenly on top of the cooked ground beef. Add the grated cheese on top.

Bake for 15 to 20 minutes. Garnish with parsley leaves, if desired.

YIELD: 6 to 8 servings

NOTE: The key here is not to let the beef dry out too much on the stovetop. As an alternative, you can add the cheese to the cauliflower when you blend it, instead of layering it on top.

Bacon Soufflé

The egg whites in this recipe create a light, fluffy soufflé texture, while the embedded bacon bits and cheese add saltiness and flavor.

INGREDIENTS

- 3 tablespoons (40 g) dry curd cottage cheese
- 1 cup (120 g) grated Cheddar cheese
- 1 cup (120 g) grated zucchini
- 3 to 4 cloves garlic, minced
- ¼ cup (20 g) cooked and finely chopped SCD-safe bacon pieces (see chart on pages 17–18)
- Salt and pepper to taste
- 2 egg whites

Preheat the oven to 350°F (180°C, or gas mark 4). Oil the bottom of a soufflé dish.

In a mixing bowl, combine the dry curd cottage cheese, Cheddar cheese, zucchini, garlic, and bacon. Add the salt and pepper to taste.

In another bowl, beat the egg whites until stiff, 3 to 5 minutes. Gently fold the egg whites into the cheese mixture.

Pour the mixture into the soufflé dish, and evenly spread it.

Bake until cooked through (a knife inserted into the center should come out clean), about 30 to 40 minutes.

YIELD: 4 to 5 servings

Simple Pork Roast

This is a quick and delicious pork recipe—the carrots and celery add a nice flavor.

INGREDIENTS

- 1 pound (455 g) boneless pork roast
- 1 tablespoon (15 ml) olive oil
- 2 cloves garlic, minced
- 1 teaspoon salt
- 1 teaspoon pepper
- 6 carrots, peeled and finely chopped
- 6 stalks celery, finely chopped

Preheat oven to 350°F (180°C, or gas mark 4).

Rub the pork with the olive oil, garlic, salt, and pepper.

Place the pork in the center of a baking dish and surround it with the carrots and celery. Cook for 1 hour, or until the juices run clear when pricked with a fork.

YIELD: 2 to 3 servings

South African Pork Patties

We created this recipe based on a South African dish called sosaties. The name sosatie is derived from sesate (skewered meat) and sate (spicy sauce). We took the base ingredients for the sosaties and added them to pork patties, which have traces of spiciness from the curry powder and sweetness from the apricots.

INGREDIENTS

- 2 tablespoons (30 ml) peanut or olive oil
- 3 cloves garlic, peeled and minced
- 1 onion, peeled and finely chopped
- 1 teaspoon Curry Powder (page 175)
- 10 SCD-safe dried apricots (see chart on pages 17–18), chopped
- 1 tablespoon (20 g) honey
- 1/4 cup (60 ml) white wine vinegar
- 1/2 cup (55 g) almond flour
- 1 pound (455 g) ground pork

Preheat the oven to 350°F (180°C, or gas mark 4). Grease an ovenproof pan.

Heat the oil in a stovetop pan, and sauté the garlic and onion over medium heat for 2 to 3 minutes. Add the curry powder and apricots and cook together for another 1 to 2 minutes. Remove the mixture from the pan and place in a large bowl.

Add the honey, vinegar, and almond flour to the bowl and combine. Finally, add the ground pork, and mix thoroughly until combined.

Make small patties out of the pork and place them in the ovenproof pan. Bake for 25 to 30 minutes. Halfway through the baking time, flip the patties over for even cooking.

Remove from the oven and drain on a plate lined with paper towels.

YIELD: 4 to 6 servings

NOTE: You can add more almond flour to the recipe if the meat base is not firm enough.

Vietnamese Pork with Shiitake Mushrooms

This pork recipe uses the Mock Fish Sauce that we created for some of our Asian-inspired dishes. The sweetness of the honey combined with the spiciness of the chiles creates a great stir-fried dish. The shiitake mushrooms add another subtle, yet distinct flavor.

INGREDIENTS

- 1 pound (455 g) boneless pork cutlet
- 2 teaspoons olive oil
- 6 cloves garlic, finely chopped
- 3 dried red chiles
- 1 tablespoon (20 g) honey
- ¼ cup (60 ml) Mock Fish Sauce (page 173)
- 3 ½ ounces (100 g) shiitake mushrooms, stems removed and finely chopped

Trim the excess fat from the pork, and cut the pork into small pieces, approximately 1 inch (2.5 cm) in length and ⅛ to ¼ inch (3 to 6 mm) in width.

Heat the olive oil in a wok over medium heat and add the garlic and whole chiles. Cook until browned, 3 to 5 minutes.

Add the chopped pork and cook for approximately 20 minutes, or until the pork is almost done. Mix in the honey and fish sauce. Turn the heat to high and cook until the sauce almost evaporates, 3 to 5 minutes.

Add the shiitake mushrooms and toss together for 1 to 2 minutes. Serve immediately.

YIELD: 4 to 6 servings

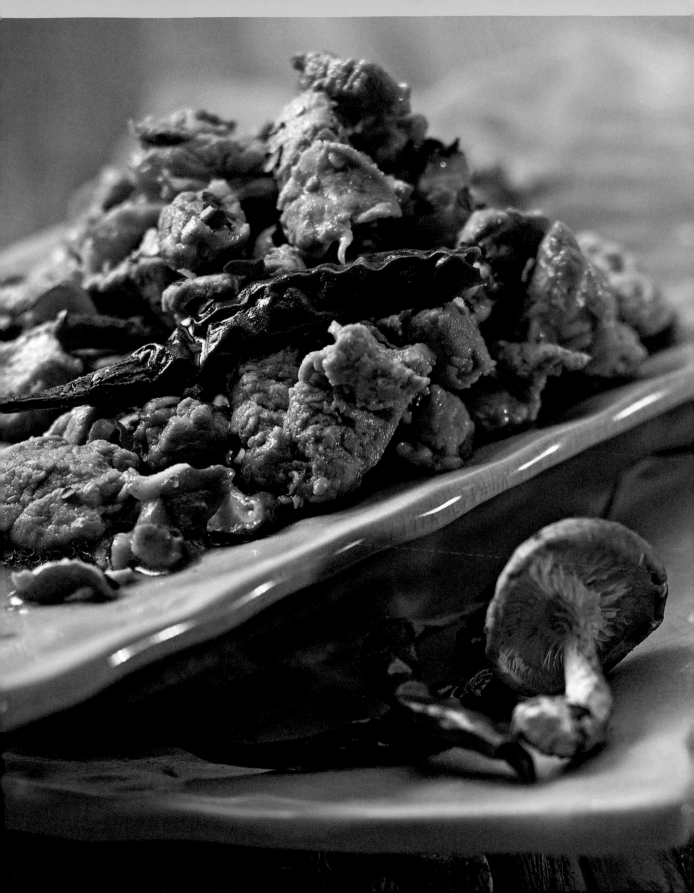

Australian Roast Lamb

Enjoy this easy-to-prepare lamb recipe. The fresh herbs add a nice touch.

INGREDIENTS

- 2-pound (910 g) leg of lamb
- 4 to 5 cloves garlic, split in half
- 1/2 to 3/4 teaspoon fresh oregano
- 1/2 to 3/4 teaspoon fresh thyme
- 1/4 teaspoon salt
- 1/4 teaspoon pepper

Preheat the oven to 350°F (180°C, or gas mark 4).

Make incisions in the lamb at evenly spaced intervals. Into these cuts, rub in the garlic, oregano, and thyme. Rub the roast with the salt and pepper.

Place the lamb on a roasting rack in the oven so that the juices can drip away while it cooks. Once it is almost cooked through (approximately 1 hour), wrap the lamb with foil so that it retains some of its juices, and roast for another 20 minutes.

YIELD: 3 to 5 servings

Tropical Lamb and Mangoes

This is an unusual combination, but the meatiness of the lamb and the sweetness of the fruit complement each other well.

INGREDIENTS

- 1/4 cup (60 g) SCD Yogurt (page 19)
- 1 lime, juiced
- 1/8 teaspoon turmeric powder
- 1/2 teaspoon salt
- 1/8 teaspoon freshly ground pepper
- 1 pound (455 g) lamb, cubed into bite-size pieces
- 1 teaspoon olive oil
- 1 large ripe mango, peeled, seeded, and cut into pieces

Combine the yogurt, lime juice, turmeric, salt, and pepper in a bowl or sealable container. Mix in the lamb pieces, and let marinate for 1 to 2 hours.

Heat the olive oil in a stovetop pan over medium heat, add the lamb, and cook for 20 to 25 minutes.

A few minutes before removing the dish from the stovetop, add the mango pieces and cook for 2 to 3 minutes, until the mango is warm.

Remove from the heat and serve immediately.

YIELD: 2 to 4 servings

NOTE: This recipe can also be made on the grill by alternating pieces of lamb and mango on a skewer.

CHAPTER 11

Vegetarian Main Dishes

On a recent trip to Lucknow, India, we walked to a nearby market with my cousins to buy vegetables for dinner. The market was dusty, but the vegetables stood out in Technicolor. (After six trips to India, the mere sight of them still makes me salivate.)

As we approached the first vendor, my cousin Anjoo's warm and jolly demeanor became more focused. I stood back while she handled the bargaining, but negotiations over carrots took longer than usual. Haggling over the cauliflower left Anjoo frowning. She never backed down on her prices, but something was amiss. Before proceeding to buy eggplant, she signaled for me to walk away from her; a few steps were not enough. I stuck out as a foreigner, causing havoc on the price haggling. Not until I was fifty yards away and around a corner would she continue shopping. Fifteen minutes later, holding bags of vegetables, we all laughed on the walk home.

Back in Mumbai, my mother-in-law, Nafisa, being older and wiser, never permits me to come vegetable shopping with her, lest I cause the same market fluctuations in her city. During my yearly visits, she spends time experimenting with her own repertoire of favorite recipes—inherited from family and friends—to make them SCD-compliant.

Eggplant Parmesan Bake

You won't miss going to the neighborhood deli anymore and staring wistfully at the daily-made eggplant parmesan. You can enjoy this version on its own, or slap it between two slices of SCD-safe bread to make your very own eggplant-parm sandwich.

INGREDIENTS

- 4 small to medium-size eggplants
- ¼ teaspoon salt
- Olive oil, for frying
- 4 to 5 medium-size tomatoes, thinly sliced
- 8 ounces (225 g) Cheddar cheese, thinly sliced, or grated
- ½ cup (20 g) basil leaves, freshly minced
- 3 cloves garlic, finely minced
- ⅓ cup (35 g) grated Parmesan cheese

Peel the eggplants and slice them into 1/8-inch-thick (3-mm) rounds. Sprinkle with salt and drain in a colander for 2 hours. Rinse and pat dry.

Preheat the oven to 375°F (190°C, or gas mark 5).

Fry the eggplant slices in olive oil in small batches and drain on paper towels. Place a layer of the eggplant slices in a 9- by 13-inch (23- by 33-cm) baking dish. Top with successive layers of tomatoes, Cheddar cheese, basil leaves, and garlic. Bake for 20 to 30 minutes.

When almost done cooking, remove from the oven, top with the Parmesan cheese, return to the oven, and bake until the cheese melts or is lightly browned.

YIELD: 6 to 8 servings

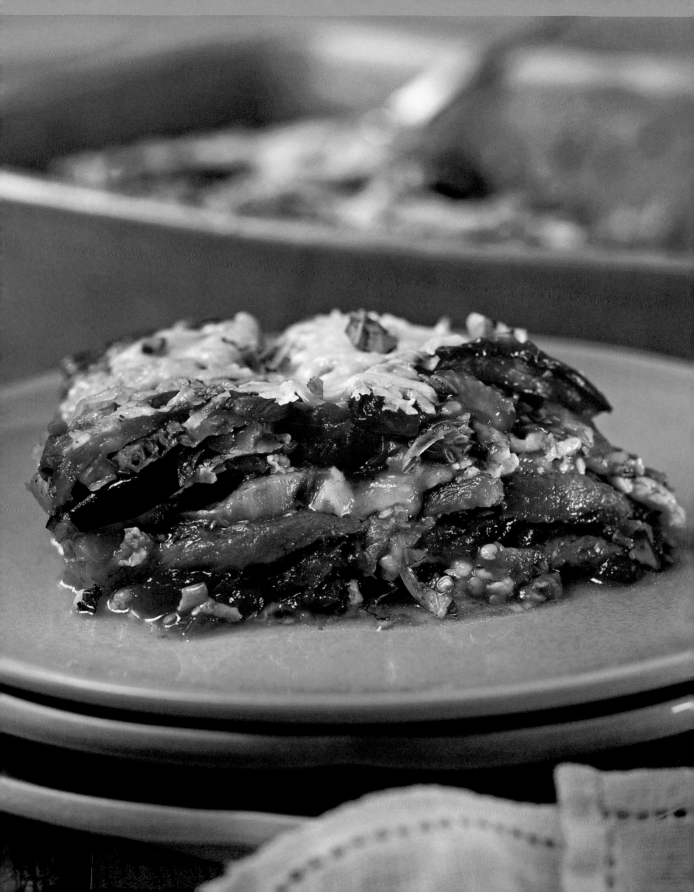

Anjoo's Aubergines

After getting married and traveling to India every one to two years, I have had a chance to reconnect with different members of my dad's family. While visiting Lucknow, a historical city where one of my dad's sisters and her family live, I was welcomed warmly into their home, and great (but failed) efforts were made to teach me Hindi every morning. More success was found in adapting recipes for the SCD; my cousin Anjoo created this eggplant recipe.

INGREDIENTS

- 2 medium-size eggplant
- 1 teaspoon salt
- 1 tablespoon (14 g) butter or Spiced Butter/Ghee (page 178)
- 5 cloves garlic, minced
- 1 large onion, chopped
- 2 teaspoons cumin powder
- 1 1/2 teaspoons coriander powder
- 1 teaspoon Curry Powder (page 175)
- Pinch of chili powder
- 4 small tomatoes, diced

Cut the eggplants into thin rounds. Salt the rounds and let them stand in a bowl for 45 minutes to drain their juices. Pat the pieces dry and cut the rounds into quarters.

In a large skillet over medium heat, heat the butter and sauté the garlic and onion for 4 to 5 minutes. Add the cumin, coriander, curry, and chili powders. Stir in the eggplant and then the tomatoes.

Cook until the eggplant is done, 25 to 30 minutes.

YIELD: 5 to 6 servings

NOTE: *Aubergine* is French for eggplant.

Sophie's Baked Almond Peppers

The capers and olives infuse this simple baked pepper recipe with a strong sensation. However, you can add different combinations of your favorite spices and vegetables to the stuffing.

INGREDIENTS

- 1 cup (110 g) almond flour
- 16 chopped black olives, pits removed
- 1 tablespoon (9 g) SCD-safe salted capers (see chart on pages 17–18)
- 2 large tomatoes, peeled and diced
- 2 large cloves garlic, mashed
- 1 tablespoon (3 g) dried oregano
- 1 tablespoon (3 g) dried thyme
- 1 tablespoon (2 g) dried basil
- 1/4 teaspoon coarsely ground black pepper
- 2 tablespoons (30 ml) olive oil, plus more for coating
- 2 tablespoons (30 ml) water
- 3 red bell peppers, seeded and cut in half

Preheat the oven to 350°F (180°C, or gas mark 4). Grease a baking tray.

Combine all the ingredients except for the red bell peppers in a food processor and blend well.

Coat the pepper halves in olive oil and place on the baking tray. Evenly divide the mixture among each pepper half. Bake for 20 to 30 minutes, or until the peppers start to char at the edges.

YIELD: 6 servings (1/2 pepper per serving)

Ravi's Mexican Burrito Wrap

My brother Ravi is the youngest in the family, but also the wisest. When he commits to an idea, he does not waver—and one of these has been becoming a vegetarian. When I asked him for a recipe, he suggested a delicious veggie wrap. The burrito below has been adapted for the SCD.

INGREDIENTS

- 3 cups (750 g) dried kidney beans*

FILLING

- 1 tablespoon (14 g) Spiced Butter/ Ghee (page 178) or butter
- ¼ teaspoon minced garlic
- 1 small onion, finely chopped
- ⅛ teaspoon red pepper flakes

- 1 tablespoon (4 g) dried or freshly chopped cilantro
- 1 zucchini, finely chopped
- 1 tomato, finely chopped
- 1 red bell pepper, seeded and finely chopped
- ½ pound (225 g) grated Cheddar cheese

WRAP

- 1 tablespoon (9 g) shelled pistachios
- 4 eggs
- 1 cup (110 g) almond flour

- 2 tablespoons (10 g) finely grated Parmesan cheese
- Butter or ghee, for cooking

To prepare the beans, cover the kidney beans with water and soak for 10 to 14 hours. During this time, rinse the beans and add fresh water if the water becomes too bubbly from the gas released from the beans.

After soaking, cook the beans by putting them in a pot of fresh water, bringing the water to a boil, and then simmering until they are soft and cooked through, 1 to 2 hours.

To prepare the filling, melt the ghee in a stovetop pan over medium heat and sauté the garlic and onion until slightly browned, 3 to 4 minutes. While they are browning, stir in the red pepper flakes and cilantro.

Next, add the zucchini, tomato, and red bell pepper, and allow them to cook until soft, 15 to 20 minutes.

When it is almost done, add the precooked kidney beans and cheese to the mixture, and stir until the cheese has melted.

To prepare the wrap, pulverize the pistachios until they are ground to a fine powder. Combine them with the eggs, almond flour, and Parmesan cheese to create the burrito wrap batter. (This batter yields 5 to 7 wraps, depending on the size of each wrap.)

Melt a bit of butter in a flat nonstick pan over low heat, and pour in some of the batter, so that it spreads thinly but evenly across the surface of the pan. Be careful not to make it very thick (the thinner the batter, the quicker the burrito cooks, and the easier it is to wrap). When one side is done cooking, flip the burrito over and cook the other side. Each side should take 2 to 4 minutes.

Evenly divide the filling among the burritos, wrap, and serve immediately.

YIELD: 5 to 7 burritos

*NOTE: Wait at least three months after symptoms have cleared before trying beans.

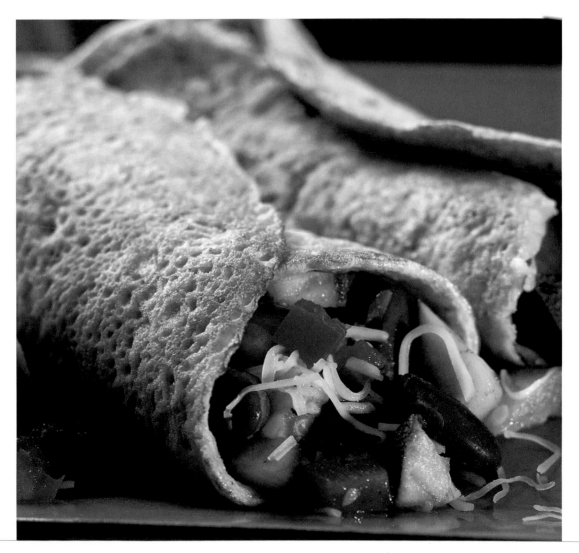

Nafisa's Traditional Dal

No matter where you travel across South Asia—whether it is into urban city centers or rural farms and villages—dal is a dependable constant during mealtimes. This particular version has been created using split peas (which are SCD-compliant), with a specific Gujarati (Western Indian) method of using the spices.

INGREDIENTS

- 2 cups (280 g) dried yellow split peas*
- 1 1/2 tablespoons (23 ml) olive oil
- 1 1/2 tablespoons (10 g) cumin seeds*
- 5 cloves garlic, finely chopped
- 2 dried New Mexico chiles
- 1 large onion, finely chopped
- 2 tomatoes, finely chopped

- 1/2 teaspoon salt
- 1/2 teaspoon cumin powder
- 1/2 teaspoon coriander powder
- 1/4 teaspoon chili powder
- 1/4 teaspoon turmeric powder
- 3/4 cup (45 g) fresh cilantro, finely chopped, for garnish

Soak the split peas in water for 10 to 14 hours. Rinse them during this period if the water they are in gets too bubbly (the peas will release gas when soaked). After soaking, drain the peas and set them aside.

Heat the olive oil in a large stovetop pot over medium heat and add the cumin seeds. Sauté for 1 to 2 minutes. Add the garlic, New Mexico chiles, and onion and sauté until brown. Add the tomatoes and cook for 5 to 10 minutes. Next, add the salt, along with the cumin, coriander, chili, and turmeric powders. Stir together to make sure the spices mix in well.

Stir the split yellow peas into the mixture, and lower the heat to a simmer. Cover the pot, and simmer until the split peas are very soft and cooked through, approximately 2 hours. Stir occasionally.

Add the fresh cilantro leaves as a garnish and serve.

YIELD: 8 to 10 servings

NOTE: *Wait at least three months after symptoms have cleared before trying lentils (including split peas) and seeds.

Baked Navy Bean Casserole

Navy beans take on the flavors of what they are cooked with—in this recipe, a bit of sweetness from the honey and tanginess from the tomatoes. The longest part of this recipe is preparing the navy beans.

INGREDIENTS

- 1 cup (200 g) dried navy beans (not canned)
- 2 tablespoons plus ½ teaspoon (32 ml) olive oil, divided
- 1 medium-size onion, diced
- 2 tomatoes, diced
- 1 tablespoon (20g) honey
- 1 teaspoon salt

Soak the beans for 10 to 14 hours, changing the water halfway through the soaking time. Rinse well.

Place the beans in a pot, cover with water, and bring to a boil. Reduce the heat and simmer for 2 hours, or until beans are cooked through and soft. Remove from the heat and rinse the beans.

Preheat the oven to 325°F (170°C, or gas mark 3).

Heat the ½ teaspoon of olive oil in a frying pan and sauté the onion until slightly brown, 4 to 5 minutes.

Combine the navy beans, cooked onion, tomatoes, honey, salt, and remaining 2 tablespoons (30 ml) olive oil in a casserole dish. Bake for 60 to 75 minutes.

YIELD: 5 to 7 servings

Sue's Spinach Cheese Puff

Like a scientist at work in a laboratory, my mother gathers, whisks, pours, and blends. She is not one of those individuals who goes by the book when she cooks—she experiments, innovates, and creates mouthwatering masterpieces of her own. Here is one of them!

INGREDIENTS

- 1 tablespoon (14 g) butter, melted
- 2 cloves garlic, minced
- 1 small onion, finely chopped
- ½ red bell pepper, diced
- 8 ounces (225 g) dry curd cottage cheese
- ½ teaspoon salt
- ¼ teaspoon black pepper
- 10 ounces (280 g) fresh spinach, stems removed and chopped
- 3 eggs
- Paprika, to taste
- grated Cheddar cheese, for garnish (optional)

Preheat the oven to 350°F (180°C, or gas mark 4). Butter a 9-inch (23-cm) square baking dish.

Melt the butter over medium heat in a stovetop pan, and add the garlic, onion, and red bell pepper. Sauté until tender, 5 to 10 minutes. Set aside.

Meanwhile, in a mixing bowl, beat together the dry curd cottage cheese, salt, and black pepper until fluffy. Stir in the chopped spinach, eggs, and the cooked stovetop mixture. Blend all ingredients until combined.

Pour into the baking dish. Sprinkle the top with paprika.

Bake for 30 to 40 minutes, or until golden brown at the edges. Right before you are about to remove the pan from the oven, if desired, sprinkle the grated cheese on the top and allow it to melt in the oven for another minute or so.

YIELD: 6 servings

West African Veggie Nut Stew

The explosion of peanut flavor in this dish turns a simple vegetarian stir-fry dish into a thick, aromatic, and spicy curry. You can vary the vegetables added to it, depending on the season or what is available.

INGREDIENTS

- 2 tablespoons (30 ml) peanut oil
- 5 cloves garlic, finely chopped
- 2 tablespoons (16 g) peeled and grated ginger
- 2 dried whole red chiles
- 1/2 tablespoon coriander powder
- 2 tablespoons (14 g) cumin powder
- 1 teaspoon cayenne pepper powder
- 1 medium-size white onion, finely chopped
- 1 small red onion, finely chopped
- 3 tomatoes, finely chopped
- 2 cups (470 ml) Basic Vegetable Stock (page 46), divided
- 4 small zucchini, finely chopped
- 2 orange bell peppers, seeded and finely chopped
- 1/2 cup (130 g) SCD-safe peanut butter (see chart on pages 17–18)

Heat the peanut oil in a wok or stovetop pan over medium heat, and sauté the garlic, ginger, and chiles with the coriander, cumin, and cayenne powders for 1 to 2 minutes.

Add both the red and white onion and cook for 4 to 5 minutes, or until browned.

Next, add the tomato and 1/2 cup (120 ml) of the vegetable stock. Bring the mixture to a boil, reduce the heat, and simmer for 10 minutes.

Stir in the zucchini and bell peppers and cook for another 20 minutes, until the peppers are soft.

Finally, mix in the remaining 1 1/2 cups (355 ml) stock and the peanut butter. Stir well to blend the peanut butter into the dish. Reduce the heat and simmer for 5 to 10 more minutes.

YIELD: 6 to 8 servings

Thin Crust Pizza

My favorite pre-SCD pizza was made at a restaurant with an old brick oven. The crust was thin enough to eat six slices in a sitting. Although we do not have a brick oven at home, this is a recipe for a delicious, thin-crust SCD pizza.

INGREDIENTS

CRUST

- 1 tablespoon plus 1 teaspoon (15 ml) oil, divided
- 2 cups (220 g) almond flour
- 2 eggs
- 1/2 cup (115 g) dry curd cottage cheese
- 1/4 teaspoon salt

TOPPING

- 2 cups (490 g) Mom's Tomato Sauce (page 172)
- 1 teaspoon oregano
- 1/4 to 3/4 (30 to 90 g) cup grated Cheddar cheese

Preheat the oven to 350°F (180°C, or gas mark 4). Grease a 9- by 13-inch (23- by 33-cm) baking dish or round pizza pan with the teaspoon of oil and set aside. To make the crust, in a bowl, combine the remaining 1 teaspoon (15 ml) olive oil with the remaining ingredients for the crust. Roll it into a ball, transfer it to the greased baking dish, and pat it down into a thin layer.

Bake in the oven for 20 minutes or until golden brown. Remove from the oven and top with the tomato sauce, oregano, and cheese. Place the dish back in the oven and bake for another 5 minutes, or until the cheese has melted.

YIELD: 4 to 6 servings

NOTE: You can layer the pizza with other toppings as desired, such as precooked vegetables or meats. Just be sure to put the cheese layer last.

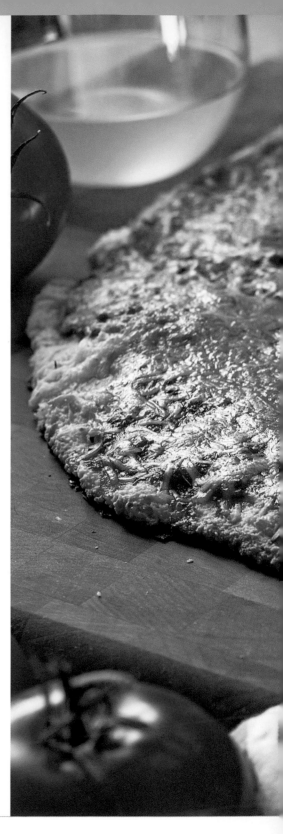

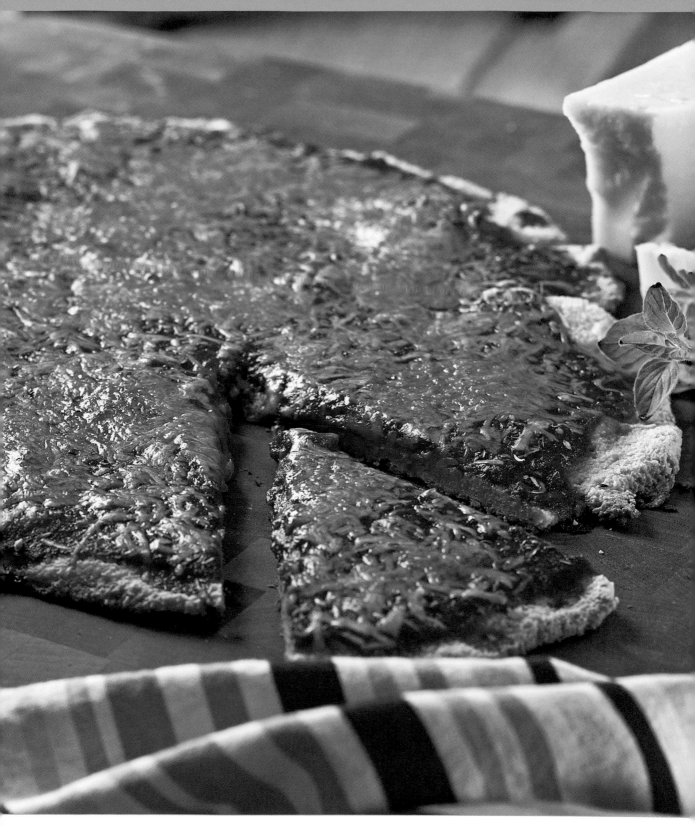

CHAPTER 12

Sauces, Dips, Dressings, and Condiments

In the winter of 2000, I decided to make pickled foods. On the kitchen counter I readied the main materials: garlic, cabbage, carrots, sea salt, and jars. It was easy: shred the cabbage, grate the carrots, bake the garlic until the skins pop off and then dice it. Mix the vegetables with salt. Place the respective vegetables in separate jars. Seal the jars with metal lids so they are airtight, and let the food ferment.

I lined up ten glass jars on the top shelves of a bookcase. Most jars were pint-size, but the sauerkraut jar, at half a gallon, towered over the others. I'd shredded more cabbage than expected. Not wanting to waste any, I filled the jar within an inch of the top. As I cleaned up the kitchen, I smiled, satisfied with a job well done.

In the middle of the night, a blast came from the living room. Dazed, I stumbled out of bed and flicked on the light. Shredded cabbage covered the wall opposite the bookcase. It also stuck to shelves, books, framed pictures, and the ceiling. And it didn't come off easily: scraping it with a fingernail barely budged the stuff. I went back to bed.

Luckily, my wife was away for another day. After an hour of moving bookshelves, attempting to rescue pictures, and scraping the wall, I realized I had no choice but to repaint. At 9 p.m., I started disposing of evidence: cleaning up the drop cloths, pulling off masking tape, putting back the ladder. When my wife arrived home the next day, it didn't take more than ten minutes before she asked: "Did you paint the room? What happened to the picture that used to be on that shelf?"

Since then I've become better at preparing food. Enjoy the condiments. No painting required.

Angie's Hollandaise Sauce

A snippet for this recipe from our friend Angie: "As an eight-year-old left with a babysitter for the weekend, I was horrified to learn that she did not know how to make hollandaise sauce when we were having artichokes for dinner. I promptly measured out the ingredients, separated the eggs, and showed her how to whisk it up on the stove. Now my three-year-old requests 'hollidaze' sauce whenever he sees artichokes in the pot."

INGREDIENTS

- 4 tablespoons (56 g) butter
- 1 tablespoon (15 ml) fresh lime juice
- 1 tablespoon (15 ml) water
- 2 egg yolks, mixed

Put the butter, lime juice, and water in a small saucepan over medium-low heat. Once the butter melts (approximately 1 minute), turn the heat down to its lowest setting. (Alternatively, you could remove the pan from the stove. This would allow the egg yolks, added in the next step, to cook in the heat generated from the hot pan.)

Add the egg yolks and stir continuously so that they mix evenly. Keep stirring so that the egg yolks do not solidify. The sauce is ready when it thickens and turns a light yellow color. This whole process should take 30 seconds to 1 minute.

Serve immediately. This recipe should be prepared right before serving, as the sauce will separate if left in the saucepan.

YIELD: 3 to 4 servings

Mom's Tomato Sauce

There is nothing like Mom's own true Italian tomato sauce. This recipe has been passed down to my mother from her mother and grandmother, and now she has given this special recipe to me.

INGREDIENTS

- 12 plum tomatoes
- 2 tablespoons (30 ml) olive oil
- 2 cloves garlic, minced
- 1 small onion, minced
- 1/2 cup (120 ml) water
- 1 cup (40 g) fresh basil leaves, chopped
- 2 tablespoons (8 g) fresh parsley
- 1 teaspoon salt
- 1/2 teaspoon black pepper

Peel, core, and dice the tomatoes. (To peel the tomatoes, immerse them in boiling water for 20 to 30 seconds and then dip them in cool water. The peels will slip off.)

In a large saucepan, heat the olive oil over medium heat and sauté the garlic and onion until tender, 4 to 5 minutes. Add the tomatoes, water, basil leaves, parsley, salt, and pepper.

Bring to a boil and then reduce the heat, simmering uncovered for 45 minutes and stirring occasionally to make sure the tomatoes are well mixed.

If you prefer a smooth sauce, allow the sauce to cool and then blend in a food processor. Refrigerate the leftover sauce for up to 5 days or freeze until needed.

YIELD: 4 to 5 cups (980 to 1225 g)

Mock Fish Sauce

This fish sauce is used in a wide variety of Thai and Southeast Asian recipes.

INGREDIENTS

- One 2-ounce (55-g) container SCD-safe anchovies, drained (see chart on pages 17–18)
- 2 cloves garlic, finely crushed
- $1/2$ teaspoon honey
- $1/4$ teaspoon salt
- 1 $1/4$ cups (295 ml) water

Combine all the ingredients in a small pan and bring to a boil. Reduce the heat to medium-low and simmer for approximately 15 minutes.

Strain the mixture to separate the anchovy and garlic pieces from the fish sauce. Reserve the strained liquid fish sauce and discard the anchovies and garlic.

Allow the sauce to cool. Refrigerate it in an airtight container. The sauce will keep for up to 2 weeks.

YIELD: $1/2$ cup (120 ml)

SCD Asian Sauce (Soy Sauce Substitute)

You can use this replacement for traditional soy sauce in a variety of Asian recipes. It is sweeter and lighter, but still has a nice punch.

INGREDIENTS

- $1/4$ cup (60 ml) red wine vinegar
- 4 tablespoons (80 g) honey
- $1/4$ teaspoon minced ginger
- $1/4$ teaspoon ground black pepper
- 2 cloves garlic, finely pounded
- 3 cups (705 ml) water
- 1 teaspoon salt

Combine all the ingredients in a small stovetop pan and cook over medium heat for 15 to 20 minutes, until reduced to $1/2$ to $2/3$ cup (120 to 155 ml).

Bottle and store in the refrigerator for up to 2 weeks.

YIELD: $1/2$ to $2/3$ cup (120 to 155 ml)

Moroccan Preserved Limes

This Moroccan recipe is used in preparing Chicken Tagine (page 111). You may also try it as a tangy accompaniment to some of the Indian recipes in this book.

INGREDIENTS

- 4 limes
- 1 quart-size mason jar, sterilized (see sterilizing instructions below)
- 1 cinnamon stick
- 3 bay leaves, cut into small pieces
- ¼ cup (72 g) salt
- 1 cup (235 ml) freshly squeezed lime juice

Cut each of the limes into 8 wedges, peel and all. Set aside.

Break the cinnamon stick into small pieces. Place a layer of salt at the bottom of the sterilized jar. Next add a layer of the lime wedges, and cover them with the bay leaves, cinnamon, and more salt. Press down on the layers to release some of the juices from the lime wedges. Continue making the layers until all the ingredients are used. Finally, pour the freshly squeezed lime juice over the layers.

Make sure that there is some air space at the top of the jar. Seal the jar tightly, and place in a cool, dry place. Shake the jar every few days, so that you distribute the ingredients within it.

You can use the lime wedges after about 2 weeks.

YIELD: 32 preserved lime wedges

NOTE: To sterilize the mason jar, wash the jar and lid with soapy water. Fill a large pot with water and submerge the jar and lid. Bring the water to a boil. Continue to boil the water for 10 minutes. Remove the jar and lid with tongs and allow to cool. (For more information, visit the National Center for Home Food Preservation at www.uga.edu/nchfp/.)

Mock Balsamic Vinegar

Use this recipe to flavor dishes such as the Wilted Mesclun with Portobello Mushrooms (page 68).

INGREDIENTS

- 3/4 cup (175 ml) red wine vinegar
- 1 cup (235 ml) red wine
- 1 tablespoon (20 g) honey

Mix all the ingredients in a saucepan, bring to a rolling boil for 3 to 5 minutes.

Reduce the heat to medium and simmer for 20 to 25 minutes. Allow the sauce to cool. Store in the refrigerator for up to 2 weeks.

YIELD: 1/2 cup (120 ml)

Curry Powder

This traditional recipe is special because all the ingredients used are in their original form. Using the whole forms of the spices also allows them to release flavors that are fresher than what you would find in a store-bought version. You can travel to the spice plantations of India to pick up the original whole spices, or alternatively, go to your local supermarket or Asian grocery store.

INGREDIENTS

- Seeds from 8 cardamom pods
- Four 1-inch (2.5-cm) cinnamon sticks
- 8 whole cloves
- 4 teaspoons whole coriander seeds
- 4 teaspoons whole cumin seeds
- 2 teaspoons whole black peppercorns
- 2 to 3 dried red chile peppers (cayenne or jalapeño), seeded

For the cardamom pods, peel off the shell casing, and pick out the black seeds. Discard the casing.

Mix all the ingredients together in a coffee grinder for 1 to 3 minutes, until you've achieved a fine, powderlike consistency.

YIELD: 1/3 cup (40 g)

Ethiopian Berberé Spice

This is a great spice blend that combines cloves, cardamom, and cinnamon with the stronger flavors of cumin, coriander, peppercorns, and chile peppers. We've used it as a base for the Ethiopian Chicken (page 114).

INGREDIENTS

- 13 dried red chile peppers
- $1/2$ teaspoon coriander seeds
- $1/2$ teaspoon cumin seeds
- 8 whole cloves
- Seeds from 10 cardamom pods
- 7 allspice berries
- $1/2$ teaspoon peppercorns
- $1/2$ teaspoon cinnamon powder, or 1 small stick cinnamon

In a small stovetop pan, dry-roast (without oil) all the ingredients until they are slightly darkened, but not burned. This should take no more than 1 to 2 minutes. (If you use cinnamon powder instead of the cinnamon stick, you do not need to add the powder to the dry-roasting process. Simply add it to the coffee grinder with the rest of the spices.)

Allow them to cool. Process all the ingredients together in a coffee grinder to achieve a powderlike consistency.

YIELD: 2 $1/3$ tablespoons (16 g)

NOTE: If you want the mixture to be less spicy, remove the seeds from the red chiles prior to dry-roasting.

SCD Coconut Milk*

Used as a base in a lot of South and Southeast Asian cooking, store-bought coconut milk frequently contains non-SCD-friendly ingredients. The process to make this homemade milk is incredibly simple, and will allow you to experiment with many of our Asian-inspired offerings.

INGREDIENTS

- 3 cups (705 ml) water
- 2 cups (140 g) dried, unsweetened, shredded coconut

Bring the water to a boil in a kettle. Place the coconut in a blender and carefully pour in the water. Mix for 3 to 4 minutes.

Strain the mixture through a fine tea strainer or cheesecloth into a bowl or jar. Discard the coconut remaining in the strainer. Store in the refrigerator and use within 2 days.

YIELD: 1 ½ to 2 cups (350 to 470 ml)

*NOTE: Wait at least six months after symptoms have cleared before trying coconut milk.

NOTE: Unsweetened dried coconut can be found at your local Asian grocery store.

Raman's Raspberry Jam

This jam is simple to make and can be spread on SCD toast, included in an afternoon snack with an SCD cookie, or eaten after dinner as a sweet accompaniment to a few scoops of SCD Yogurt (page 19).

INGREDIENTS

- 1 tablespoon (14 g) butter
- 1 tablespoon (20 g) honey
- 7 ounces (195 g) fresh raspberries*

In a small stovetop pan, melt the butter over medium heat. Slowly add the honey, stirring it into the butter until it dissolves. Add the fresh raspberries and allow all the ingredients to simmer together for 5 to 10 minutes, until thickened.

Store in the refrigerator in an airtight container. This will keep for 2 to 3 weeks.

YIELD: 1 cup (320 g)

*NOTE: Wait at least three months after symptoms have cleared before trying raspberries.

Spiced Butter/Ghee

In India, ghee (clarified butter) is cooked and used in many homes. It has its roots in thousands of years of historical traditions, myths, and ceremonies. We added a touch of spiciness to the mainstream clarified butter recipe so that when you use this ghee as an ingredient in some of our other dishes, like the Ethiopian Chicken (page 114) or Beef Vindaloo (page 141), it imparts a wonderful flavor.

INGREDIENTS

- 2 pounds (910 g) unsalted butter, cut into small pieces
- 1 small onion, coarsely chopped
- 10 cloves garlic, minced
- 1 1/2 tablespoons (12 g) peeled and grated ginger
- 3 whole cloves
- 1 teaspoon turmeric powder
- 1/4 teaspoon cardamom powder
- 1/2 teaspoon cinnamon powder
- 1/4 teaspoon ground nutmeg
- 1/4 teaspoon chili powder

In a large saucepan, melt the butter slowly over medium heat; do not let it brown. Bring the butter to a boil and stir in the onion, garlic, ginger, cloves, and turmeric, cardamom, cinnamon, nutmeg, and chili powders. Reduce the heat and simmer uncovered and undisturbed for 45 minutes. The milk solids on the bottom of the pan should become golden brown, and the butter on top will be transparent.

Slowly pour the clear liquid into a bowl, straining it through a cheesecloth. Discard the milk solids. Make sure there are no additional solids left in the liquid.

Pour the liquid ghee into a jar. Cover tightly, and store in the refrigerator for up to 2 months.

YIELD: 1 1/4 pounds (570 g)

Sophie's Artichoke Tapenade

The artichoke gets its name from the Arabic "ardi shauk" meaning "ground thorn." The "choke" is the outer leaves of the plant that are inedible and usually discarded, while the "heart" is the soft inner core.

INGREDIENTS

- 4 artichoke hearts
- 1 clove garlic, mashed
- 3 tablespoons (45 ml) olive oil
- 1/2 to 3/4 teaspoon salt, or more to taste
- 1/4 teaspoon black pepper, or more to taste
- Juice from 1/2 lime

Steam the artichokes in a stovetop steamer until soft, 15 to 20 minutes. Peel off and discard the outer leaves of the artichokes (harder parts), and save the softer, inner hearts for the tapenade. Combine the hearts with the garlic, olive oil, salt, and pepper in a blender and blend until smooth, 3 to 5 minutes. Stir in the lime juice and add more salt and pepper if necessary.

YIELD: 1 1/2 to 2 cups (340 to 450 g)

Cilantro Dip/Spread

This recipe may accompany some of the South Asian dishes that are in this book, as a cooling but flavorful condiment. It also makes a great spread to go with the savory Curry Crackers (page 38).

INGREDIENTS

- 6 tablespoons (80 g) Yogurt Cheese (page 182)
- 1 clove garlic, minced
- 1/8 teaspoon chili powder
- 1/4 teaspoon salt
- 1 teaspoon dried cilantro
- 1/4 teaspoon cumin powder
- 1 teaspoon lime juice

Mix all the ingredients together in a small bowl.

Serve immediately, or refrigerate in a covered container for up to 3 days.

YIELD: 3/8 to 1/2 cup (90 to 125 g)

Roasted Red Pepper Relish

The first secret behind this recipe is roasting the peppers just right, so that they do not burn to a crisp, but soften and sweeten. The second one is allowing the roasted red peppers to marinate well in the olive oil.

INGREDIENTS

- 2 red bell peppers, whole
- 2 orange bell peppers, whole
- 6 tablespoons (90 ml) olive oil
- 2 cloves garlic, mashed
- 1/4 teaspoon salt
- 1/4 teaspoon black pepper

Preheat the oven to 400°F (200°C, or gas mark 6) or set to broil. Roast the red and orange bell peppers in the oven until the skins blacken and the peppers soften. Remove and cool. Peel off the skins, cut in half, and remove the seeds.

Finely dice the peppers, and mix in the olive oil and garlic. Add the salt and pepper. Place in a sterilized jar (see instructions for sterilizing jars on page 174) and allow to marinate for at least 1 day before serving.

YIELD: 1 1/2 cups (270 g)

Thanksgiving Stuffing

Thanksgiving in our family was always about coming to the dinner table at my parents' home to enjoy an amazing spread, put together by my mom, Sue Ann. It is during this American celebration that she outdoes herself the most—from the succulent turkey to an array of appetizers, side dishes, and desserts.

INGREDIENTS

- 2 spring onions, finely chopped
- 3 apricots, finely chopped
- 3 tablespoons (27 g) shelled pistachios, finely chopped
- 1 cup (100 g) pecans, finely chopped
- ¼ cup (15 g) parsley, finely chopped
- ¾ teaspoon salt
- ¼ teaspoon pepper
- 1 ½ to 2 cups (75 to 100 g) crumbled SCD-safe bread (see chart on pages 17–18)

Mix all the ingredients together in a bowl. Serve with Thanksgiving turkey.

You can heat this stuffing, or serve it as is.

YIELD: 3 to 4 cups (150 to 200 g)

NOTE: Crumbled pizza crust (page 168) works well as a substitute for the bread.

Yogurt Cheese

Yogurt cheese has a thick, creamy consistency, which lends itself to making dips, frostings, and spreads.

INGREDIENTS

- 2 cups (490 g) SCD Yogurt (page 19)

Yogurt cheese is made by straining yogurt. Layer a strainer or colander with cheesecloth and pour the yogurt on top.

Underneath, place a bowl or other container to catch the liquid whey. Cover and refrigerate for 6 to 8 hours. (Instead of a strainer/colander, you can also purchase a commercial yogurt cheese maker.)

You can discard the liquid whey that strains through—the yogurt cheese is the part that remains in the strainer.

YIELD: 1 cup (245 g)

NOTE: To thicken the yogurt cheese, strain it for a longer period of time, up to 24 hours.

CHAPTER 13

Sweet Baked Goods and Other Desserts

The party involved two cakes and forty people crammed into our modest Brooklyn apartment. In the hours before being served, cake #1 drew the most attention: large, chocolate, and purchased from a heavily patronized neighborhood bakery.

When the cutting hour arrived, cake #2 emerged from the refrigerator: small, frosted, and SCD-friendly. Upon the initial cutting, I received a slice of the SCD cake. However, I made the mistake of drifting to the center of the room and being drawn into conversation. It couldn't have been more than fifteen minutes, but I never received a second piece. Word had spread and the SCD cake disappeared before cake #1 reached the halfway point.

On many special occasions, the phenomenon of the "amazing-disappearing-SCD-cake" has repeated itself. Since then, I make sure to sneak away extra pieces, hiding them in the back of the freezer until the guests leave.

More recently, my brother and his girlfriend have made a ritual of getting together with us to play our favorite board game, but they really just come to bake and eat batches of SCD-friendly cookies and treats.

Almond Puffs

This recipe comes from Portugal, and it is a delicious, dairy-free dessert. When we pulled it out of the oven, it was extremely airy inside, and melted in our mouths. So get those forearms working—the more you whisk those egg whites, the fluffier and more tantalizing these will be!

INGREDIENTS

- 12 eggs, divided
- 1 cup (320 g) honey
- 1/4 cup (60 ml) hot water
- 3 cups (330 g) almond flour
- 1/8 teaspoon cardamom powder
- 1/8 teaspoon vanilla extract

Preheat the oven to 300°F (150°C, or gas mark 2). Butter a 9- by 13-inch (23- by 33-cm) baking dish.

Take 6 of the eggs and separate the egg whites from the yolks. Set the yolks aside. Beat the egg whites until stiff, about 10 minutes. Set aside.

Mix together the honey and hot water to create a diluted syrup. Add the 6 remaining eggs, 6 reserved yolks, cardamom powder, vanilla, and almond flour to the syrup. Stir to combine. Slowly fold in the stiffly beaten egg whites.

Transfer the mixture to the buttered baking dish and bake for 20 to 30 minutes, or until golden. The consistency of the baked dish should be fluffy and light.

Cool and cut into small squares.

YIELD: Twenty-five 2-inch (5-cm) squares

Gretel's Gingerbread Cookies

We have all read the universal Grimm fairy tale, Hansel and Gretel, in which two children wandering through the forest come upon a witch's house made of gingerbread. Imagine an SCD version of this story that would appeal to kids on the diet—they would dream of a house made of Almond Puffs (at left), cinnamon squares (page 192), and gingerbread cookies, as in this recipe below.

INGREDIENTS

- 8 tablespoons (112 g) butter, melted
- 1 egg
- 1 teaspoon water
- 1/4 cup (80 g) honey
- 1/2 teaspoon allspice powder
- 2 teaspoons ginger powder
- 1/2 teaspoon clove powder
- 1/2 teaspoon cinnamon powder
- 1/8 teaspoon peeled and grated fresh ginger
- 1 teaspoon baking soda
- 3 cups (330 g) almond flour, or more as needed

Preheat the oven to 350°F (180°C, or gas mark 4). Grease a cookie sheet.

Mix all the ingredients together in a bowl, until the dough is dry enough and not sticky to work with. Add more almond flour, if necessary.

On the cookie sheet, form 1 1/2- to 2-inch (4- to 5-cm) circular mounds with the dough and press down to flatten into a cookie shape.

Bake for 10 to 15 minutes, or until the edges turn golden.

YIELD: 40 to 45 cookies

NOTE: This is modified from a recipe that was contributed to the www.scdrecipe.com website (which the author created and maintains) by Diane from Florida. Thanks, Diane!

Lemon Cookies

The risky part about this recipe is that you can eat the batter as well as the final product. One guest of ours once decided to do just that, so now we hide the batter preparation during any visits!

INGREDIENTS

- 4 tablespoons (56 g) butter, melted
- 1/3 cup (105 g) honey
- 1 teaspoon lemon zest
- 1/8 teaspoon baking soda
- 2 1/4 cups (1025 g) almond flour

Preheat the oven to 350°F (180°C, or gas mark 4). Grease a cookie sheet.

Mix all the ingredients together in a bowl. The batter should be moist. Roll the batter into small, 1/2-inch balls. Place the balls on the greased cookie sheet, evenly spaced apart. Press down and flatten.

Bake until golden brown, 10 to 15 minutes. Allow to cool.

YIELD: 25 to 30 cookies

Uncle Jim's Pignole Cookies

My Uncle Jim was a true gentleman. He fought in WWII, yet when we talked with him, he was down-to-earth and humble about his experiences. He was a steady and dependable sort of guy—the only time he succumbed to excesses was when my Aunt Betty would make him his favorite pignole cookies.

INGREDIENTS

- 1 cup (135 g) pine nuts
- 1/3 cup (105 g) honey
- 4 tablespoons (55 g) butter, melted
- 2 1/2 cups (275 g) almond flour
- 1/2 teaspoon SCD-safe almond extract (see chart on pages 17–18)
- 4 egg whites, beaten stiff

Preheat the oven to 350°F (180°C, or gas mark 4). Grease a cookie sheet.

Mix all the ingredients, except the egg whites, together in a large bowl. When they are well blended, slowly fold in the egg whites. The dough should be firm, but moist. Make 1/2-inch balls of dough, and drop onto the greased cookie sheet, spacing them evenly apart.

Bake until the cookies turn golden brown, 10 to 15 minutes.

YIELD: 25 to 30 cookies

Transylvanian Hazelnut Cookies

The hazelnuts in these simple cookies add a nice touch to the almond flour that we normally use to create SCD baked goods. The prevalence of hazelnuts in baking in modern-day Romania (which is most familiar in fairy-tale lore as the home of Dracula) makes us think that these cookies would be especially indulgent as a late-night treat while watching a good horror or mystery movie.

INGREDIENTS

DOUGH

- 1 cup (150 g) whole hazelnuts
- 1 1/4 cups (140 g) almond flour
- 1/2 teaspoon baking soda
- 2 tablespoons (28 g) butter, melted
- 2 1/2 tablespoons (38 ml) water

GLAZE

- 1 tablespoon (14 g) butter
- 1 tablespoon (20 g) honey
- 1/8 teaspoon cinnamon

Preheat the oven to 375°F (190°C, or gas mark 5). Grease a cookie sheet.

To make the dough, finely grind the hazelnuts in a food processor. In a mixing bowl, combine the blended hazelnuts and the remaining dough ingredients. The dough should be quite firm, although the consistency of the hazelnuts might make it a bit crumbly.

To make the glaze, heat together the butter, honey, and cinnamon in a small stovetop pan. Mix until the butter melts and remove from the heat.

Create individual cookies with the mixture. Press down to make as flat as possible. Bake for 10 to 15 minutes, or until the edges are golden brown. Remove from the oven, and brush the glaze onto the tops of the cookies. Place back in the oven for another 1 to 2 minutes, or until the glaze has melted into the cookies.

Remove from the oven and let cool. Store in an airtight container.

YIELD: 10 to 15 cookies

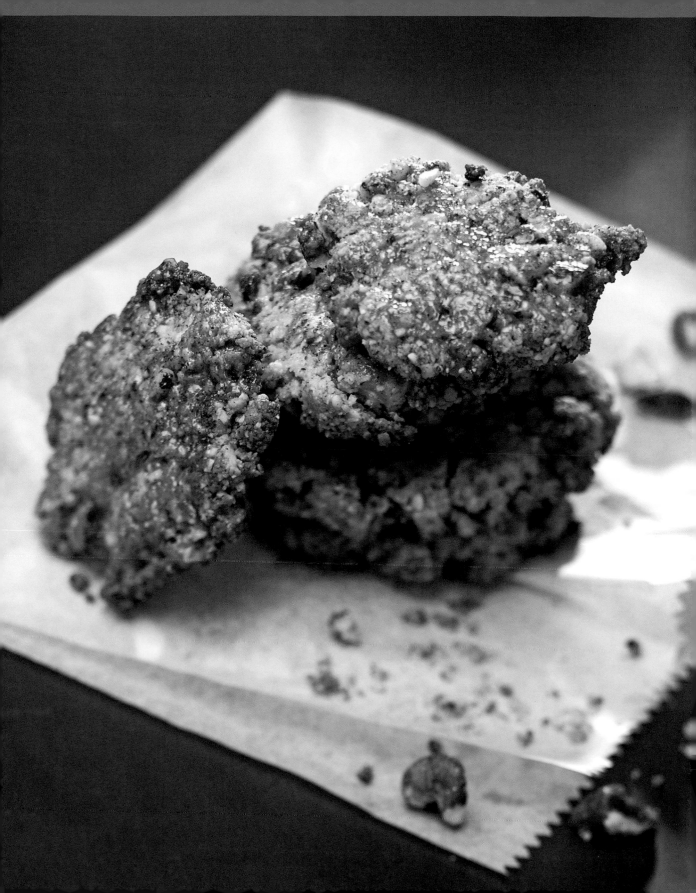

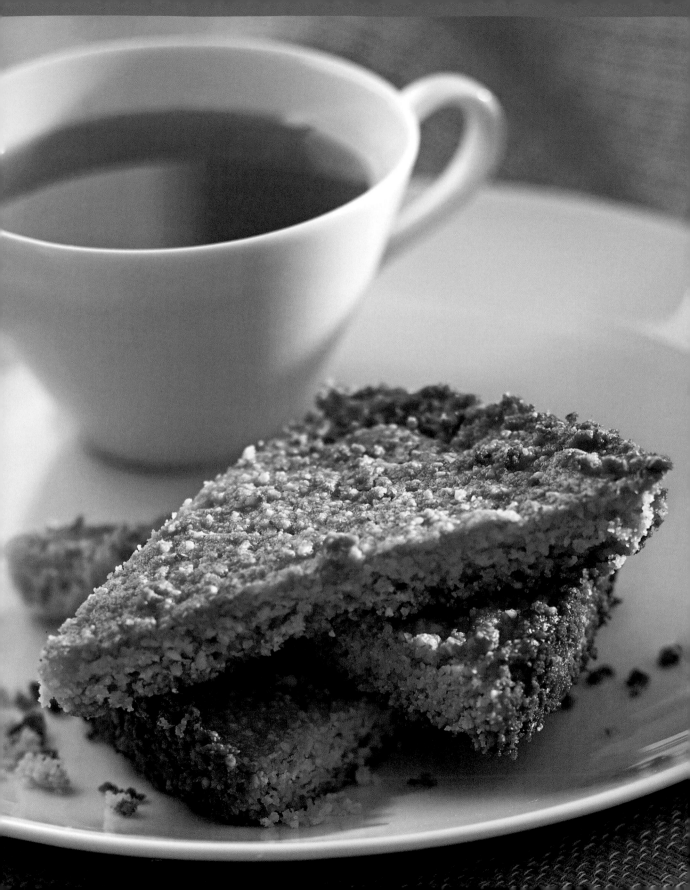

Scottish Shortbread

Shortbread gets its name from the "shortening" used in the recipe, which, in our case, refers to the butter. This classic biscuit has roots in Scotland, but it is popular elsewhere in Europe, as well as in the United States. This recipe is unbelievably good. You can't even tell that it is an SCD shortbread!

INGREDIENTS

- 2 cups (220 g) almond flour
- 6 tablespoons (85 g) butter, melted
- 2 1/2 tablespoons (50 g) honey

Preheat the oven to 350°F (180°C, or gas mark 4). Have on hand a 9- or 12-inch (23- or 30-cm) circular pan.

Mix all the ingredients together in a bowl. The dough should be greasy enough from the butter that you do not need to butter the baking pan.

Press the shortbread dough into the pan, and bake for 15 to 20 minutes, until golden brown.

Let it cool in the pan, then cut into wedges and store at room temperature in an airtight container.

YIELD: 8 wedges

NOTE: Puncture the batter in the pan with the tip of a fork before baking, to allow the batter to cook evenly through.

Quyên's Cinnamon Squares

Our friend Quyên loves SCD baked goods, to the point that it has become a mini-tradition to make cinnamon squares together when we meet.

INGREDIENTS

- 3 cups (330 g) almond flour
- 1 pinch baking soda
- 4 tablespoons (55 g) butter, melted
- 1/2 teaspoon cardamom powder
- 3/4 teaspoon cinnamon powder
- 1/4 teaspoon vanilla extract
- 1/4 cup (80 g) honey
- 2 egg whites, beaten stiff

Preheat the oven to 350°F (180°C, or gas mark 4).

Combine all the ingredients together in a mixing bowl, except for the egg whites.

Mix thoroughly, and then fold in the beaten egg whites. Pour into a 9- by 13-inch (23- by 33-cm) ovenproof dish and bake until a knife inserted into the center comes out clean, approximately 15 minutes. Cut into squares.

YIELD: 20 to 24 squares

Pear Compote

This is a great side for main dishes or desserts. The natural sweetness of the pears is subtle and delicious. It goes especially well with the Parmesan and Walnut Crusted Chicken (page 117).

INGREDIENTS

- 2 large pears
- 2 tablespoons (28 g) butter

Peel the pears, and finely chop them.

Heat the butter in a saucepan, and add the pears. Cook on medium-low heat. Cover the pan with a lid, but not completely, so that there is room for some moisture to escape.

Stir occasionally, until the pears are softened and cooked through, approximately 10 minutes. Mash the pears with a fork or hand-held mixer, so that they become smooth.

YIELD: 1 1/2 to 2 cups (370 to 490 g)

Christmas Cake with Vanilla Frosting

Christmas cakes differ all over the world, with the condition that most have some type of fruit. This past holiday, I was presented with the following SCD Christmas cake.

INGREDIENTS

CAKE

- 3 1/2 cups (385 g) almond flour
- 1/2 teaspoon baking soda
- 1/2 teaspoon cinnamon powder
- 1/4 teaspoon clove powder
- 1/4 teaspoon allspice powder
- 1/4 teaspoon nutmeg powder
- 3 eggs
- 1/2 cup (115 g) dry curd cottage cheese
- 1/3 cup (105 g) honey
- 4 tablespoons (55 g) butter, melted
- 1/2 cup (75 g) golden raisins
- 8 SCD-safe dried apricots (see chart on pages 17–18), cut into small pieces

VANILLA FROSTING

- 5 teaspoons Yogurt Cheese (page 182)
- 1 1/2 teaspoons honey
- 1/4 teaspoon vanilla extract
- 1/4 teaspoon cinnamon powder

Preheat the oven to 350°F (180°C, or gas mark 4). Butter a 9- by 13-inch (22- by 33-cm) baking dish.

To make the cake, combine all the cake ingredients thoroughly in a food processor. Spread the batter evenly in the pan. Bake for 30 to 45 minutes, or until a knife inserted into the center comes out clean. Remove from the oven and let cool.

To make the frosting, in a small bowl, whip together the frosting ingredients, until they have reached a smooth consistency.

After the cake has cooled, spread the frosting on top. If you add the frosting while the cake is still hot, it will get absorbed into the cake because of the heat, so make sure it has fully cooled.

YIELD: 15 to 20 servings

Pineapple Upside-Down Cake

*This American classic has been created for the SCD with fresh pineapples.
Do not use the canned variety, or if you do, make sure that there are no
preservatives or sugars added to them. We prefer a fresh, ripe pineapple,
as the juices from the slices seep into the batter and flavor it nicely.*

INGREDIENTS

BATTER

- 2 cups (220 g) almond flour, or more as needed
- 3 eggs
- 4 tablespoons (55 g) butter, melted
- 1/2 cup (160 g) honey
- 3/4 teaspoon vanilla extract
- 1/4 teaspoon cinnamon powder

- 1/2 pound (230 g) fresh pineapple, thinly sliced

Preheat the oven to 350°F (180°C, or gas mark 4). Grease a 8- or 9-inch (20- or
23-cm) circular baking dish.

To make the batter, mix the batter ingredients in a food processor until smooth.
Add more almond flour if necessary to make sure the batter is not too thin.

Layer the pineapple slices on the bottom of the baking dish, and then pour in
the cake batter and spread it evenly in the pan.

Bake the cake for 30 to 40 minutes, or until a toothpick inserted into the center
comes out clean.

YIELD: 15 to 20 servings

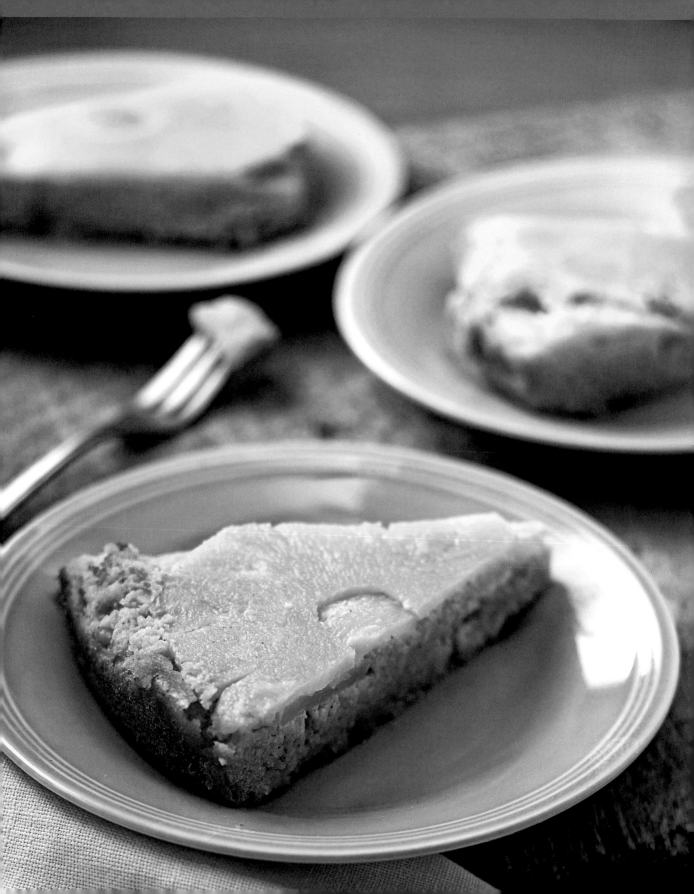

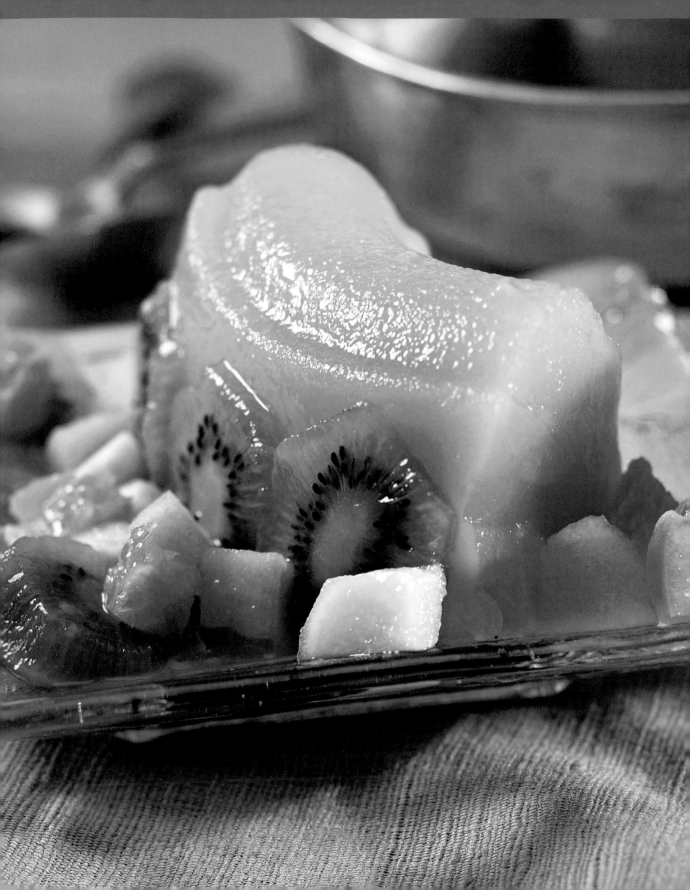

Orange JELL-O with Fruit

This dessert has universal appeal—children love the JELL-O and their parents love the healthy fruits involved. It requires no baking and lasts for several days.

INGREDIENTS

- 3 cups (705 ml) freshly squeezed orange juice
- Four 1-ounce (28-g) packets unflavored gelatin
- 1 cup (235 ml) hot water
- 1 teaspoon honey
- 1 orange, peeled and diced into small pieces
- 1 apple, peeled and diced into small pieces
- 1 pear, peeled and diced into small pieces
- 1 kiwifruit, peeled and cut into thin slices

If you have a JELL-O mold, you may use it, or use a flat-bottomed container. Make sure the container you use is deep enough to hold the 4 cups of liquid and the fruit.

In a large bowl, mix the orange juice and the gelatin. Stir the hot water into the orange-gelatin mixture. Add the honey, and keep stirring until the gelatin has dissolved.

Add the orange, apple, and pear pieces, and allow them to settle into the gelatin mixture. Pour the mixture into the container or JELLO-O mold.

Gently place the sliced kiwis on the top, being careful not to put too much pressure so that they float on top of the JELL-O and do not sink to the bottom. Alternatively, you can line the kiwi slices along the edge of the container and then pour the mixture in.

Cover with plastic wrap or the container's top, and place in refrigerator for at least 3 hours, or until the JELL-O is firm.

Enjoy!

YIELD: 8 to 10 servings

Raspberry Granita/Sorbet

When you are sitting out on your porch in the summer, with a good book, your dog lazily stretched out on the grass, this fruit-based sorbet is a refreshing indulgence.

INGREDIENTS

- 6 pints (1800 g) frozen raspberries*
- 4 cups (940 ml) water, divided
- 1 orange, juiced
- ½ cup (160 g) honey
- Mint sprigs or fresh raspberries,* for garnish

Purée the raspberries in a food processor or blender until smooth. Add 1 ½ cups (350 ml) of the water to the mixture while blending (otherwise the purée gets too thick).

Pass the processed mixture through a sieve so that you only get the raspberry purée, and the seeds are left behind.

Place the strained mixture in a stovetop pan. Add the orange juice, honey, and remaining 2 ½ cups (590 ml) water. Bring to a simmer, stirring constantly. Remove the pan from the stovetop, and allow to cool to room temperature.

Stir the mixture thoroughly, pour into a container, and freeze for approximately 12 hours. Stir it every few hours to redistribute the slush. The mixture should get firm, but still be a bit slushy. After 12 hours, re-blend the mixture in a food processor, until it is smooth and frothy.

Return the mixture to the freezer container, and place in the freezer overnight or until firm.

When ready to serve, scrape the granita with a fork to fluff it up. Add a sprig of mint or a few fresh raspberries for garnish.

YIELD: 6 to 8 servings

*****NOTE:** Wait at least three months after symptoms have cleared before trying raspberries.

Mango Ice Cream

This recipe is a cinch to make. You can serve it with fresh mangoes to your guests after dinner, or just scoop out a few spoonfuls for yourself on a hot summer night.

INGREDIENTS

- 2 cups (490 g) SCD Yogurt (page 19)
- 2 tablespoons (18 g) shelled pistachio nuts
- 1/4 cup (80 g) honey
- 2 mangoes, peeled and cut into pieces

Blend all the ingredients in a blender until smooth. Place in the freezer until frozen.

YIELD: 4 to 6 servings

NOTE: You can also use an ice cream maker for this recipe.

Banana Nut Date Bread

The dates, walnuts, and bananas blend together to create a sweet, nutty indulgence. The vanilla extract promises an additional hint of sweetness. Enjoy this on its own or with a scoop of SCD Yogurt (page 19).

INGREDIENTS

- 1/2 cup (160 g) honey
- 1/4 cup (60 ml) vegetable oil
- 1 egg
- 1 teaspoon vanilla extract
- 1 medium-size ripe banana, mashed
- 2 tablespoons (28 g) butter, melted
- 3 cups (330 g) almond flour
- 1 teaspoon baking soda
- 1/2 teaspoon salt
- 1 cup (175 g) chopped dates
- 1/2 cup (50 g) chopped walnuts

Preheat the oven to 350°F (180°C, or gas mark 4). Butter a 9- by 13-inch (23- by 33-cm) baking dish.

Blend all the ingredients together in a food processor. Depending on how you prefer the texture of the dates and walnuts, you can add them into the mixture and blend them well, or add them later if you like them chunkier.

Pour the batter into the baking dish. Bake for 25 to 30 minutes, or until a knife inserted into the center comes out clean.

YIELD: Fifteen 2-inch (5-cm) squares

Nonnie's Thanksgiving Pie

There is nothing that my wife Nilou looks forward to more at Thanksgiving than my grandmother Nonnie's pie.

INGREDIENTS

CRUST

- 1 1/2 cups (165 g) almond flour
- 1 egg
- 1/8 teaspoon vanilla extract
- 1 tablespoon (14 g) butter, melted
- 1/8 teaspoon cardamon powder
- 1/8 teaspoon clove powder
- 1/2 tablespoon honey

FILLING

- One 1- to 1 1/2-pound fresh butternut squash
- 1/4 cup (85 g) honey
- 1/3 cup (75 g) dry curd cottage cheese
- 1/4 teaspoon cinnamon powder
- 1/4 teaspoon clove powder
- 3 egg whites, beaten stiff

Preheat the oven to 325°F (170°C, or gas mark 3). Butter an 8" (20 cm) Pyrex (glass) baking dish. To make the crust, mix all the crust ingredients together in a bowl. The dough should be moist, but not too runny or soft. Place in the baking dish and press down so that the dough covers the base and the sides of the baking dish. Make it as thin as possible. Set the crust dish aside.

To make the filling, peel the butternut squash, cut it in half, scoop out the seeds, and dice the squash into small 1" (2.5 cm) pieces. Steam the squash until soft, approximately 20–25 minutes, and puree in a food processor. Measure out 1 1/2 cups (340 g) pureed squash, and blend this with the honey, dry curd cottage cheese, cinnamon, and clove powder in the food processor until well mixed. Slowly fold the egg whites into the blended mixture. Pour the filling into a separate baking dish.

Place the pie-filling dish in the oven and cook for 30 minutes. Then place the pie crust dish into the oven, and let both cook separately for 10 minutes. Remove both the dishes from the oven, and pour the semi-cooked pie filling into the crust dish. Place back in oven and cook together for 10–15 minutes. Remove from oven and allow to cool.

YIELD: 8 to 10 servings

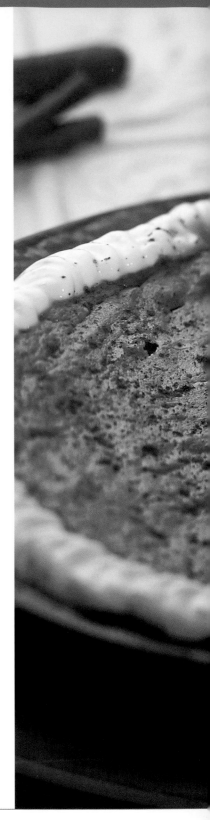

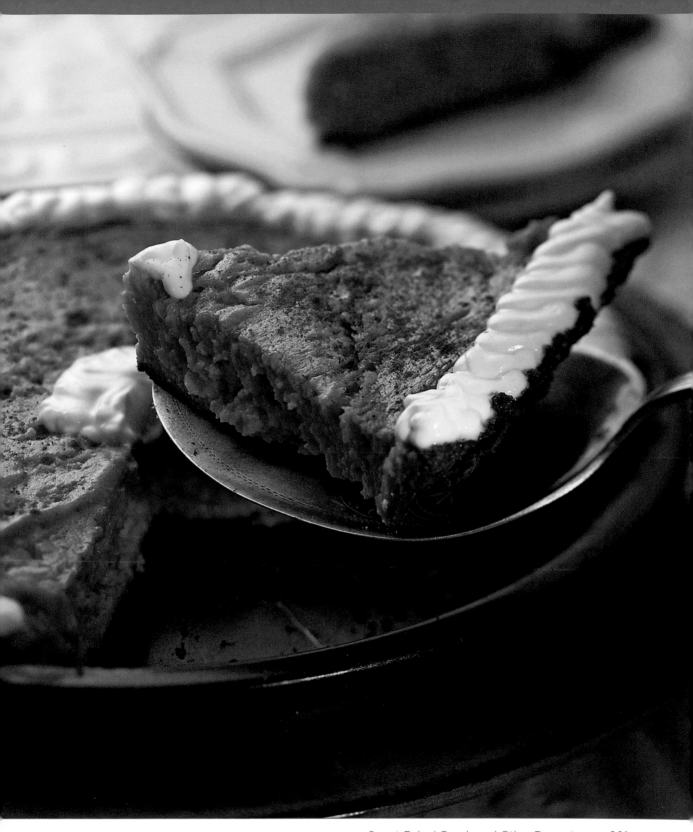

Strawberries with Balsamic Vinegar and Cracked Black Pepper

We tried this recipe on our friends, Ori and Dina, who were visiting overnight. They looked confused when we listed the ingredients, but they took a second serving once they tasted it. The blending of tart vinegar and spicy pepper mapped onto the sweet strawberries is extraordinary.

INGREDIENTS

- 1 pound (455 g) strawberries
- 4 teaspoons Mock Balsamic Vinegar (page 175)
- Cracked black pepper, as desired

Wash the strawberries and remove the tops. Cut them into slices and set on a dessert plate so that they are laid out evenly and not heaped on top of each other.

Drizzle the balsamic vinegar over the strawberries. Grind some black pepper on top. Serve.

YIELD: 4 servings

NOTE: Add a dollop of SCD Yogurt (page 19) to each serving if you'd like.

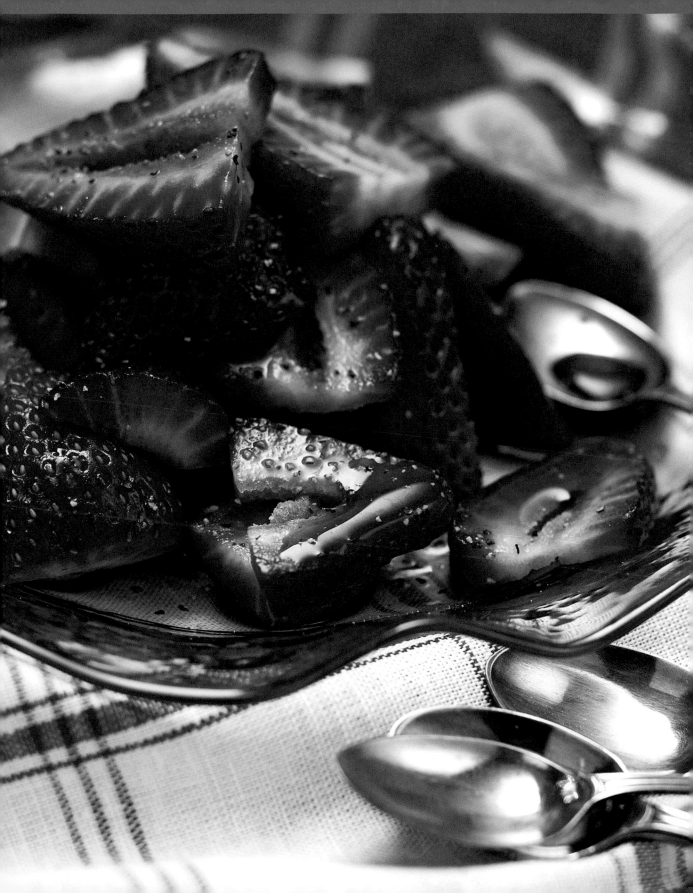

CHAPTER 14

Drinks

A friend living overseas would always ask the same question when visiting: "Are you still eating the same breakfast? Chopping your apples in the morning?"

For many years, the answer was "yes." But now I've discovered the blender and made a move to smoothies. I open the fridge, throw in some dry curd cottage cheese, SCD Yogurt, an apple or a banana, and push the "on" button! Voilà! One giant glass of breakfast! Sometimes I throw in pecans, raisins, or maybe a teaspoon of honey.

However, if you're thinking of making smoothies, there's a danger. The drink tastes so good that you'll tilt your head back and tip the glass nearly upside down to get the last drop. The upper rim of the glass may touch your face, leaving a white, chalk-like streak running across your nose—it's all part of the early morning smoothie initiation ritual. Focused on the taste, you may not notice the food mark.

But it's obvious to other people—the neighbors, the U.P.S. delivery man, random strangers on the street, and especially your partner—who may or may not tell you that it's there.

Beet Juice

This beet juice has a great color as well as taste.

INGREDIENTS

- 2 large beets
- 6 cups (1410 ml) water
- 2 limes, juiced
- 1 1/2 teaspoons honey
- 1/4 teaspoon salt
- 1 1/2 teaspoons cumin powder
- 2 cups (470 ml) club soda, or carbonated water
- Lime slices, for garnish

Peel the beets and coarsely chop them into pieces. Combine the water and beets in a stovetop pan and bring to a boil. Reduce the heat and simmer until the beet pieces are cooked through and soft, 30 to 45 minutes.

Allow it to cool, and then blend the beets in a blender. Add the lime juice, honey, salt, and cumin powder. The consistency will be quite thick. This process will yield about 4 cups (940 ml) of concentrate.

Before serving, for every 2/3 cup (155 ml) of juice, mix in 1/3 cup (78 ml) of club soda. Stir well, and garnish with a lime slice.

YIELD: 6 cups (1410 ml)

Fruit Juice Blend

This juice blend takes a tangy direction with the addition of the cumin powder.

INGREDIENTS

- 1 banana, peeled and cut into pieces
- 2 oranges, peeled and cut into pieces
- 1 pear, peeled, cored, and cut into pieces
- 3/4 to 1 tablespoon (15 to 20 g) honey
- 1/4 cup (60 ml) water
- 1/16 to 1/8 teaspoon cumin powder

Combine all the ingredients in a blender. Pour into a tall glass and serve immediately.

YIELD: 1 serving

NOTE: You can try variations of this recipe with other fruits, such as apples, grapefruit, etc.

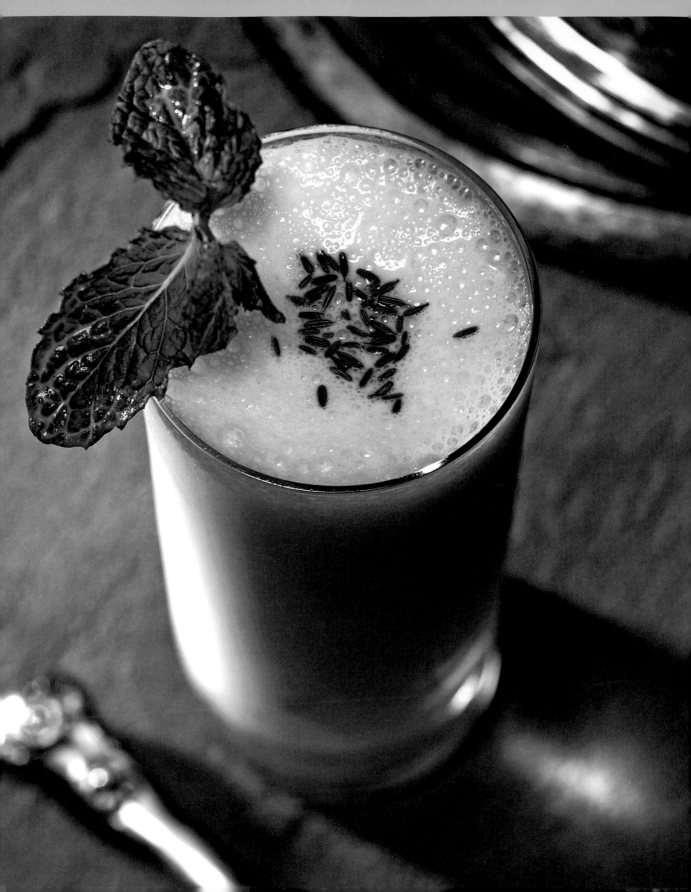

Jeera Lassi

This traditional yogurt drink is an Indian specialty that is cooling and refreshing in the summer heat.

INGREDIENTS

- ½ teaspoon whole cumin seeds*
- 1 cup (245 g) SCD Yogurt (page 19)
- ¾ cup (175 ml) water
- Salt and pepper to taste
- Ice (optional)
- 2 to 3 mint leaves, for garnish

Dry-roast the cumin seeds by cooking them in a small pan (without oil) over medium heat. Stir them until they turn a darker brown (this should take no longer than 1 minute), and immediately remove from heat. Be sure not to burn them. Set aside a few of the seeds for garnish, if desired.

In a blender, combine the remaining cumin seeds, yogurt, water, salt, and pepper.

Pour into a glass and add ice cubes, if desired. Garnish with mint leaves and reserved cumin seeds and serve.

YIELD: One 10-ounce (285 ml) glass

***NOTE:** Wait at least three months after symptoms have cleared before trying seeds.

Minty Limeade *(pictured at right)*

Our mint-infused limeade has Mediterranean roots, but it is enjoyed through-out the world.

INGREDIENTS

- 4 limes, juiced
- ¼ to ⅓ cup (85 to 115 g) honey
- 2 tablespoons (12 g) fresh mint leaves, or as desired
- 2 cups (470 ml) water
- Ice, as desired
- Lime slices, for garnish (optional)

Combine all the ingredients except the ice in a blender. Once mixed, add the ice and pulse for a few more seconds until the ice is crushed. Garnish with lime slices, if desired. Pour into tall glasses and serve immediately.

YIELD: 3 cups (705 ml)

NOTE: Add more water if you prefer your limeade more diluted, or more honey if you prefer it sweeter. If you do not like the mint blended into the drink, you can add it afterward.

Papaya-Lime Fizz

This quick drink does not take more than a couple of minutes to make and is tart and tangy. It makes a great summer drink.

INGREDIENTS

- 1 cup (140 g) sliced papaya
- 1 ½ to 3 cups (350 to 705 ml) club soda, or carbonated water
- 1 lime, juiced

Combine all the ingredients together in a blender. Pour into tall glasses and serve.

YIELD: 1 to 2 servings

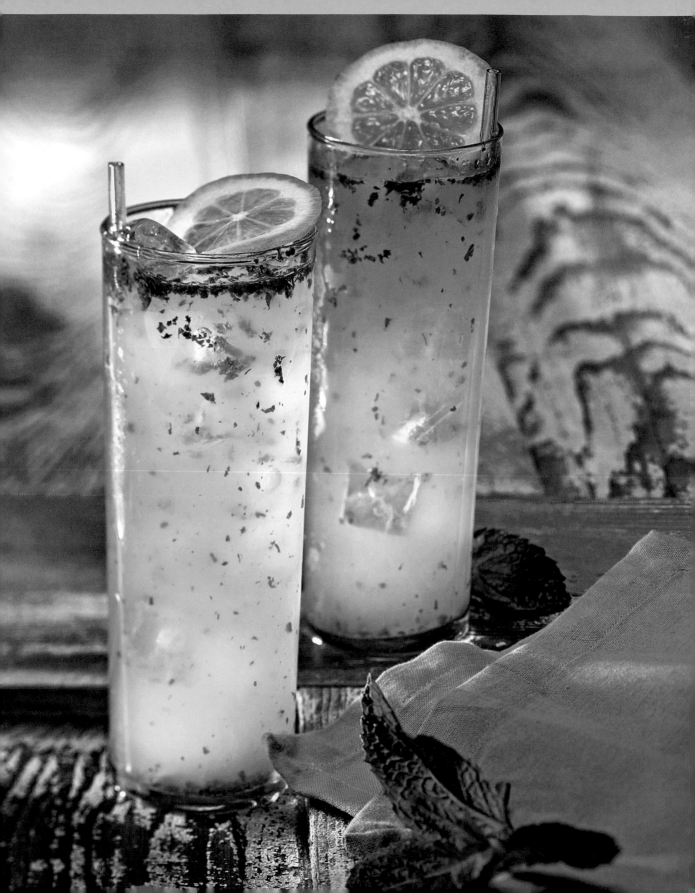

Tangy Tomato Juice

The chile in this drink recipe turns a plain tomato juice into a spirited, spicy beverage that's sure to wake up your taste buds.

INGREDIENTS

- 4 large tomatoes, coarsely chopped
- 1 small serrano chile, seeded and finely chopped
- 1 teaspoon salt
- 1/2 teaspoon pepper
- Cilantro sprigs, for garnish

Thoroughly combine the tomatoes, chile, salt, and pepper in a blender, and then strain to remove the seeds and excess pulp.

Pour into glasses and garnish with a cilantro spring before serving.

YIELD: 3 1/4 cups (765 ml)

Hot Ginger Tea

This infusion is soothing for when you are feeling sick, or simply on a wintry night.

INGREDIENTS

- 1/2 cup (50 g) fresh ginger slices, peeled
- 2 cups (470 ml) water
- 4 whole cloves
- 4 whole cardamom pods
- 1 small cinnamon stick
- 1/2 teaspoon lime juice
- 1 1/2 teaspoons honey

Bring the ginger, water, cloves, cardamom, and cinnamon to a boil in a stovetop pan. Reduce the heat, cover, and simmer for 10 minutes.

Add the lime juice and honey and simmer for another 2 to 3 minutes. Strain the tea, and serve immediately.

YIELD: 2 cups (470 ml)

Resources

The following references provide further information regarding the Specific Carbohydrate Diet. When starting the diet, it's helpful to join one of the online mailing lists described on www.breakingtheviciouscycle.info or www.pecanbread.com. In addition, these sites have links to further references.

Websites

www.breakingtheviciouscycle.info
The official *Breaking the Vicious Cycle* website. This site contains definitive information for the SCD diet.

www.scdrecipe.com
Created by the author, this site lists hundreds of SCD recipes, originally compiled from the SCD mailing lists. In addition to an organized collection of recipes by category, this site contains SCD news updates and other relevant information.

www.lucyskitchenshop.com
Lucy Rosset has created a website that offers items relevant to the SCD diet, including yogurt makers, yogurt starter, almond flour, and other products.

www.pecanbread.com
This site describes treating autism with the SCD, including the science behind the diet as well as a section on transitioning a child to the SCD. In addition, there are instructions on how to sign up for active online support groups.

www.scdiet.org
This site contains relevant information for those following the diet, including SCD resources, and community and FAQ sections, among others.

Other Websites:
www.scdiet.com
www.gottschallcenter.com
www.digestivewellness.com
www.scdiet.net
www.scdbakery.com

Books

Breaking the Vicious Cycle
By Elaine Gottschall
This is the primary book on the SCD.

Colitis & Me: A Story of Recovery
By Raman Prasad
This memoir chronicles the author's struggle to overcome IBD—a lifelong illness marked by bloody intestines, cramping, and fear—while simultaneously facing life's exciting questions, possibilities, and challenges.

Fast Food Nation
By Eric Schlosser
Entertaining and fact-filled, this book explores different aspects of the fast food industry, much of which also applies to packaged foods.

The History of a Crime against the Food Law: The Amazing Story of the National Food and Drugs Law Intended to Protect the Health of the People; Perverted to Protect Adulteration of Foods
By Harvey W. Wylie
Written in 1929 by the head of the Division of Chemistry of the U.S. Department of Agriculture, predecessor of the Food and Drug Administration, this book chronicles the fight for U.S. food laws. It includes the story of how the 1906 Pure Food Law came into being—and was later dismantled. Although not fast reading, the book is quite interesting. (There's even congressional testimony on how chemically created dextrose/glucose should not be sold as "corn sirup [syrup]," as it would lead to too much available sugar and a decline in public health.)

Management of Celiac Disease
By Sidney V. Haas and Merrill P. Haas
The original book on the SCD; availability is often limited to medical school libraries.

What to Eat
By Marion Nestle
This book examines in-depth food available in the supermarket. It provides a much greater understanding about buying food, from fish and meats to fruits and vegetables.

Acknowledgments

We would like to thank the following people:

Elaine Gottschall, whose tireless dedication in furthering SCD knowledge allowed others to regain health and good spirits once again. Thank you, too, to Elaine's daughter, Judy Herod, and our SCD compatriot Lucy Rossett, for spending valuable hours reviewing the manuscript.

The Fair Winds Press team, who have given us the opportunity to create this cookbook—specifically Cara Connors and Amanda Waddell, who both worked tirelessly to pull together the manuscript; and Rosalind Wanke and the creative staff who were involved in the food photography and visual design.

Thank you to the Moochhala family, especially our mom Nafisa, and sisters Sophie and Zenobia, who have contributed precious time and energy in creating part of this collection.

Thank you to the Prasad family and relatives, for their unwavering enthusiasm and invaluable time spent sharing family recipes with us, especially our mom Sue Ann.

Thank you to our friends, who have been SCD creators, tasters, and testers throughout this process and beyond.

And finally, thank you to all those in the SCD community who have provided us with unending support and enthusiasm.

About the Authors

Raman Prasad was first diagnosed with ulcerative colitis at the age of seventeen. His health steadily deteriorated in the years that followed, resulting in several hospital stays and various health complications. It was during this time that he came across Elaine Gottschall's book, *Breaking the Vicious Cycle*, which outlined the Specific Carbohydrate Diet (SCD) and the science behind it for putting inflammatory bowel disease (IBD), celiac disease, and diverticulitis in remission.

Raman has followed the SCD successfully for more than ten years with the help of his wife, **Niloufer Moochhala**, which has resulted in a happy return to good health and a normal life. Inspired by his recovery, the couple created an online recipe database for the SCD community and established www.scdrecipe.com in 1998. Over the past decade, the website has grown to include more than 500 recipes, as well as other relevant information about the diet.

A native of North Haven, Connecticut, Raman (who is of Indian and Italian-American heritage), is also the author of the self-published memoir *Colitis & Me: A Story of Recovery* and the SCD cookbook *Adventures in the Family Kitchen,* which combines traditional Italian-American and Indian recipes from the couple's respective families (Niloufer was born and raised in Mumbai, India).

Together, the two have traveled widely in an effort to create a global kitchen within the SCD repertoire. From indulging in chicken curry in the ancient Indian city of Udaipur to feasting on Spanish tapas in old Barcelona, their mission has been to taste and re-create SCD-safe recipes offered by other cultures and traditions and thereby expand the diversity of the diet.

They live in Boston with their dog, Serif.

Index of Dairy-Free Recipes

When using the SCD for autism, dairy products should be avoided for at least the first six months. The following recipes do not contain dairy products.

NOTE: Please consult your doctor before using the diet for autism. You can find support through www.pecanbread.com.

Index